Suffering Narratives of Older Adults

In *Suffering Narratives of Older Adults*, Mary Beth Quaranta Morrissey turns to the traditions of phenomenology, humanistic psychology and social work to provide an in-depth exploration of the deep structure of the suffering experience. She draws upon the notion of Maternal holding to develop an original construct of *Maternal Affordances* – the ground of possibility for human development, agency and relational practices. Morrissey's conceptual analysis is based on the life narratives of several elders receiving chronic care in facility environments.

Creating new fields of communication for patients, their family members and health professionals in processes of reflection and shared decision making, this book builds on knowledge about suffering to help guide ethical action in preventing and relieving chronic pain and improving systems of care. It offers a phenomenological approach to understanding the Maternal as a primary domain of moral experience in serious illness and suffering, and implications for policy, practice and research. A series of applied chapters, looking at individual experiences of suffering and care experiences, present critical areas of ethical inquiry, including:

- pain and suffering;
- Maternal-relational ethics;
- evaluation and moral deliberation about care options;
- decision making and moral agency; and
- end-of-life experiences of care.

Exploring how an ecological relational perspective grounded in phenomenology may provide fruitful alternatives to traditional frameworks in bioethics, this is an important contribution to the ongoing development of an ecological ethic of care. It will be of interest to scholars and students of bioethics and phenomenological methods in the health and human services, as well as practitioners in the field.

Mary Beth Quaranta Morrissey, PhD, MPH, JD, is a Fellow of the Global Healthcare Innovation Management Center, and the Program Director of the Post-Masters Healthcare Management Certificate Program in Public Health, Palliative Care and Long-Term Care, Fordham Schools of Business, New York, USA.

Routledge Advances in the Medical Humanities

New titles
Medicine, Health and the Arts
Approaches to the Medical Humanities
Edited by
Victoria Bates, Alan Bleakley and Sam Goodman

Suffering Narratives of Older Adults
A Phenomenological Approach to Serious illness, Chronic Pain, Recovery and Maternal Care
Mary Beth Morrissey

Forthcoming titles
Doing Collaborative Arts-based Research for Social Justice
A Guide
Victoria Foster

Learning Disability
Past, Present and Future
C. F. Goodey

The Experience of Institutionalisation
Social Exclusion, Stigma and Loss of Identity
Jane Hubert

Digital Stories in Health and Social Policy
Listening to marginalized voices
Nicole Matthews and Naomi Sunderland

Medical Humanities and Medical Education
How the Medical Humanities Can Shape Better Doctors
Alan Bleakley

Suffering Narratives of Older Adults

A Phenomenological Approach to Serious Illness, Chronic Pain, Recovery and Maternal Care

Mary Beth Quaranta Morrissey

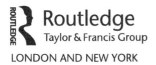

Routledge
Taylor & Francis Group

LONDON AND NEW YORK

First published 2015 by Routledge

2 Park Square, Milton Park, Abingdon, Oxon OX14 4RN

711 Third Avenue, New York, NY 10017, USA

Routledge is an imprint of the Taylor & Francis Group, an informa business

First issued in paperback 2017

British Library Cataloguing-in-Publication Data
A catalogue record for this book is available from the British Library

Library of Congress Cataloging-in-Publication Data
A catalog record has been requested for this book

ISBN: 978-0-415-85479-5 (hbk)
ISBN: 978-1-138-70321-6 (pbk)

Typeset in Times
by Saxon Graphics Ltd, Derby

To my mother, Mary Ann

Contents

Foreword

There is a growing recognition of the staggering social problems that loom in the graying of the baby boom generation. The population of seniors in the United States is projected to more than double over the next 40 years, rising from 35 million in 2000 to over 88 million by 2050. At that time, one in five Americans will be age 65 or older. Those 80 and above will be the most populous age group in the country—32.5 million or 7.4 percent of the population. America's chronic and long-term care systems are patchwork, and they are insufficient to meet the challenges that these demographic trends will create. Can our society make better provision for those who built it a generation ago? Basic social decency and respect for the humanity and dignity of those in the shadows and the twilight of their lives, today and in the future, hang in the balance.

Undergoing treatment for serious chronic illness and frailty in a long-term care setting is dislocating, very much like entering an alien world in which one must suspend one's normal rights, freedoms, expectations, and routines. It involves the replacement of one's persona by a very different institutional identity and role. Even if an elderly person receives long-term care in the home, this social dislocation can occur.

Moreover, regardless of setting, long-term care often has to grapple with pain, which must be controlled, and it must come to grips with suffering, which must be assuaged. While the patient undergoes the suffering, exposure, and helplessness of submitting to the "bed and body work" of long-term care, he or she is socially and morally indulged by those to whom the caregiving has been entrusted. This experience can precipitate a crisis of self-identity and meaning. Paradoxically it can cause an alienation from one's past just when it is precisely that past that one is desperate to regain.

The foremost challenge of an aging society, I take it, is the retrieval—or perhaps the reconstruction—of meaning: What is the nature and meaning of old age? How does it fit in the overall voyage of life? Can there be a cultural skein weaving the living generations together in a complementary and supplementary, rather than an antagonistic, fashion? Central to these and related questions of meaning are the notions of rights and relationships, notions that are profoundly shaped and defined by the—not always consistently meshing—frameworks of medicine and law, of public policy and caregiving practice, of ethics and economics.

From what perspective can we best understand suffering in the last chapter of life and an ethic of care which is both rights-oriented and relational? Where should we look for insight into the experience of suffering and the meaning of the caring response that suffering calls forth?

In *Suffering Narratives of Older Adults*, Mary Beth Morrissey turns to a highly creative and nuanced application of the traditions of philosophical phenomenology and humanistic psychology for answers to these questions. In so doing, she provides an in-depth exploration of the deep structure of the suffering experience. In her account, the aspects of relief and palliation, while vitally important, cede center stage to aspects of continuing self-actualization and effective agency. She uses the notion of maternal caring—a fundamental impulse to nurture that lies at the root of the experience of suffering when it is truncated—to develop an original construct. Maternal caring is grounded in a relational practice in which the agency of those who receive care, and the agency of those who provide it, work together in a kind of symbiosis. Morrissey's conceptual analysis is based on the life narratives of several residents of a long-term care facility; her construction of these narratives grows out of extended qualitative interviews. This book is an important contribution to the ongoing development of an ecological ethic of care. Her wide reading and mastery of philosophical phenomenology and humanistic psychology are impressive, but I am struck even more by the contribution that this book makes to an important paradigm shift now underway in the field of bioethics.

Bioethics is not simply a specialized version of disciplinary moral philosophy. It is an interdisciplinary field that is based on a particular way of designing the interconnection between theory and practice. Bioethics at its best engages with the actually existing values, norms, and cultural belief systems that form the context for human behavior. It is a sensitive barometer of the social context within which the human experience and meaning of health and illness take shape. Bioethics moves fluidly from the most intimate personal needs and experiences to the broadest social, systemic, and policy questions. Pain makes policy vivid and compelling; suffering makes systems come alive as tangible social agents rather than as intellectual constructs or abstractions.

I think there is no doubt that bioethics has succeeded over the years in injecting a higher standard of ethical propriety and self-consciousness into medicine and health care on both the levels of clinical practice and public policy. Nonetheless, the discourse and social influence of bioethics has not powerfully challenged or threatened the biomedical establishment, including the operative assumptions and patterns of long-term care. It is true that bioethics today is becoming more self-reflective and critically aware of the conceptual limitations of its own discourse, but this is a relatively recent trend, prompted often by the work of feminists, philosophers working out of non-analytic traditions (such as phenomenology), social scientists, and others who are able to adopt an external stance on mainstream bioethics. *Suffering Narratives of Older Adults* makes a distinguished contribution to this critical reflectiveness in the field.

In my view, the main blind spot of bioethics thus far has been its abstract individualism. It has at both the clinical and the policy level regularly lacked an adequate contextual understanding in terms of historical change, political economy, and power. And in terms of individual agency and experience, it has failed to develop an adequate way of comprehending the self in relational or "ecological" terms. Informing most work in bioethics is an idea of culture and society, tradition, solidarity, and community as instrumental handmaidens in the service of autonomous, independent interests, desires, and negative rights. Relationality on this view is only the stage setting, the scenery behind the enactment of unencumbered individual choice and action.

What is needed today is a shift in orientation—a movement of tectonic plates in our moral imagination and caring practices, so to speak—to produce a new conceptual foundation for long-term care and palliative care, understood broadly as the response to suffering at any stage of life. It is this shift from individualistic interests to a relational and communicative perspective and orientation that is so clearly exemplified in Morrissey's work. This perspective sees the situation of the seriously chronically ill and impaired person as a social situation as much as a biological one. The process of receiving and giving care takes place within a system of interdependencies and a network of shared meanings. The relational orientation combines respect for developmental personhood with recognition of the inherent dignity of all human beings and their need for care, presence, and relief of suffering—in a word, their deep connection to the maternal dimensions of human experience. It is based on the insight that human beings are not self-sufficient or self-sovereign individuals but are interdependent, ecological selves. The intention of long-term care—its telos or what it aims to realize—is to support aging well and living well by navigating relationships and meanings, memories past, meanings present, and hopes for the future intact through the shoals of crisis.

Morrissey writes in order to bring high quality standards and a depth of moral imagination to long-term care. She brings to the foreground the complex nexus of social and cultural relations among human beings, and her interview-based narratives of individual residents reveal their extraordinarily diverse and powerful affective and communicative capacities.

The hour is upon us when it is essential to *reorient* our predominant cultural understandings of suffering among the frail elderly. This is both a scientific and a philosophical undertaking. This involves enacting policies and practices based on an understanding of the good of human flourishing, at any age and functional level: an understanding of the good that is necessarily rooted in robust scientific investigation and inference, but also premised on the enduring experiences and traditions of humankind, as we can know them from historical and anthropological study. There has been a strong tendency in bioethics to starkly separate public considerations of policy from conceptions of the good. And there has also been a tendency in bioethics to think mainly of utilitarian individualism, with its notions of preference satisfaction and consumptive, hedonic interests, as the only reasonable conception of the human good appropriate in a secular society. A bioethics that is adequate to the task of responding ethically to suffering in an aging society requires more than this.

Deployed as Morrissey does, phenomenology has the capacity to reveal a better conception of the human good than utilitarianism provides. For Morrissey agency and personhood are constituted, not *in spite of* connections and commitments linking self to others, but *in and through* these connections and commitments. Enacting one's life is a process that develops a self-identity built out of ongoing practices (what she calls "affordances") that exemplify the creative and aesthetic dimensions of a humanness. Her relational conception of personhood contains a counter-vision to notions of alienation and the objectification of the human Other. It reflects the contextual, socially, and symbolically mediated nature of self-identity and agency. It seeks to reconcile individual self-direction (autonomy) with interdependency, nurture, and community.

It is certainly striking that so much work in bioethics has focused on individual autonomy and on concerns about professional or social paternalism. It is often expedient to frame important ethical issues, in the clinical encounter between physician and patient for instance, in this way, but doing so incorporates certain ontological and normative views about society that are unnoticed and uncritically accepted. For example, it often seems to be assumed that we should begin our ethical consideration with an assumption of non-interference and the liberty of the individual to pursue independent interests. Then the burden of ethical argument is to provide reasons why the needs and interests of others ought to be taken into account, perhaps curtailing independence in favor of mutuality. Why not turn this on its head and start with a presumption of moral relationship and reasons of connection and interdependency, and then put the onus on finding exceptional grounds that permit individuals to override the presumptive ethical obligations inherent in their condition of social and moral membership?

Societies and communities are too uncritically assumed in many bioethics discussions to be mere backdrops for individual life and agency, viewed as conditions we use and exploit, not as places where we live and have our being. Values are not viewed in any kind of historical or cultural context, nor are they seen as things that predate or constitute who we are. In *Suffering Narratives of Older Adults*, Mary Beth Morrissey helps to rectify bioethics in that regard and to set us on a more fruitful path of reflection and moral caring. This is a brave book and an important service.

Bruce Jennings
Director of Bioethics at the Center for Humans and Nature
Senior Advisor and Fellow at The Hastings Center

Acknowledgments

I am considerably blessed to be the recipient of the kind of empathic caring, mentoring and nurturing that I describe in my book and that is so desperately needed for those who are suffering. It is with appreciation and love that I acknowledge those who have helped me reach the point where I am today.

First and foremost, I acknowledge my dear and beloved mother, *Mary Ann Quaranta*, who provided me with a very loving home from my earliest years through my mature adulthood – making possible my growth and development and the fruition of my interests. By "home," I mean not only a physical place but the fertile ground for my intellectual, emotional, and spiritual life. It was always my great joy to engage in conversation with my mother because she was so unusually open, receptive, and attentive, and made her presence keenly felt in ways that were highly supportive and enabling. She introduced me to very progressive ideas as early as my yet-undeveloped mind was able to embrace them, stimulating my interest in as many things in the world as were possible to afford me, and gifting me with a restlessness that was never to be quieted. I dedicate this book to my mother, *Mary Ann*.

I express my deepest gratitude to all the members of my family as they have supported my work throughout my career, beginning with my husband Ed, who has made it possible for me to pursue intensively my studies, research, and writing. My five lovely children—Mary Breda, Kathleen, Kerianne, Teddy, and John—have also been a constant source of support, each in her/his own way. To Kerianne, I owe a special debt of gratitude for her unwavering devotion and facilitation of my every need during my doctoral studies and in this period of my development as an early career scholar. I continue to be amazed and delighted by the depth and breadth of insight shown by Kerianne—who has studied research herself while pursuing her bachelor's degree in social work, and especially her interest in and understanding of my study of phenomenology and utilization of phenomenological methods.

In my professional life, I have benefited from the guidance and wisdom of many outstanding scholars, many of whom I have encountered in my studies at Fordham University—my second home, where I earned my undergraduate degree, as well as my JD and PhD. I first thank my college English professor Mark Caldwell, who inspired and supported my early interests in writing and college thesis work on Hegel and Virginia Woolf. I was also privileged as a college student to study Hegel with Quentin Lauer, and more recently as a doctoral student, to sit in some of John Drummond's lectures on moral phenomenology.

I pause to recognize in a special way my doctoral studies' mentors at Fordham. I remain deeply indebted to Meredith Hanson, Director of the Doctoral Program in Social Work and my mentor in the Graduate School of Social Service (GSS). Meredith gave me the relational support and complete freedom to explore, express and develop my ideas throughout my time in the doctoral program. In his role as chair of my dissertation committee, he guided the development of my proposal and the timely completion of my study right up through my successful defense. Meredith also understood my fierce independence, as well as my sensitivity and vulnerability. I thank him for facilitating my very positive experience in the doctoral program at Fordham.

I acknowledge GSS professor emerita Nancy Boyd Webb, who has written prolifically on families and bereavement, and GSS professors Cathy Berkman and Virginia Strand, outstanding researchers and scholars who have supported the development of my scientific interests.

Finally, I come to my mentor Fred Wertz, professor and past chair of the Psychology Department at Fordham, and the methodologist for my dissertation. I thank Fred for helping me to transform my thinking in my middle life. Over the nearly seven years that I have worked with Fred, our encounters have never failed to be unsettling, providing a continuity of engagement in diverse types of provocative and exciting intellectual inquiries and reflections. In the truest sense, Fred epitomizes all that I describe in this book about the maternal dimensions of existence and its affordances. My readers may appreciate more fully the impact that my formal introduction to phenomenology through Fred, and my exposure to its philosophic foundations, have had on my development as a scholar in both challenging the foundations of my knowledge and opening up new horizons and vistas in my intellectual life. Fred introduced me to the rich history and contexts of humanism and human science, and to the French phenomenologists— Emmanuel Levinas, Gabriel Marcel and Maurice Merleau-Ponty. For these gifts, as well as for his capacity to navigate our human contexts of uncertainty and difference, I remain eternally grateful to Fred and highly value his brilliance, scholarship, receptivity and friendship.

Moving outside of the Fordham community, in my more than decade-long relationship with my colleague Bruce Jennings, who is a prominent bioethicist and highly respected scholar in many circles, I have had the opportunity to discuss my ideas freely and receive Bruce's generous and erudite feedback in the context of many projects on which we have collaborated. Bruce has had a guiding influence in shaping my work. Although I am not sure Bruce would call himself a phenomenologist, his orientation is phenomenological and he understands why phenomenology is so meaningful to social ecologies and social practices. I am honored to call Bruce my trusted colleague, mentor and friend.

In keeping with my rootedness in Jesuit tradition, I have found it equally rewarding at this mid-stage of my career to experience a warm collegiality with

Michael Barber, a highly esteemed scholar. I have had the honor and pleasure of getting to know Michael over the last few years through the Interdisciplinary Coalition of North American Phenomenologists, and aspire to appreciate more fully the depth and range of his scholarship. Michael, who is Dean of the School of Arts and Sciences at St. Louis University, has influenced me not only through his writing, but also through his humility and generosity in helping me understand some of the most challenging questions and subjects in phenomenological philosophy. I cherish his collegiality and friendship.

There are three individuals to whom I owe abundant thanks for their editing support in facilitating the completion of this project. They are John D. Stahl, English professor and family friend; Judy Mendell, colleague in the doctoral program at Fordham and with whom I have developed a rewarding friendship; and Allison Peltzman, whose grandmother, Bea, was a very dear family friend and my one and only Jewish mother until her very last days. Bea's empathy and care are reflected in the continuity of our friendship into the next generations.

I do wish to acknowledge the several care facilities that permitted me to conduct research at their sites. I apologize that I am not free to recognize them by name due to my constraints in protecting the anonymity and privacy of my study participants. However, I express admiration and respect for those who are serving the very sick, the frail and the dying in these care facilities, and the loving care that I have witnessed being provided by staff at every level of institutional life.

Introduction

This book is a phenomenological account of suffering among seriously ill older adults drawn from the research investigations I have conducted at care facilities during the last four years. My motivation for undertaking this research project, which has brought me face-to-face with suffering elders, resides in scientific and ethical interests in describing and deepening understanding of suffering experience, and how suffering is socially constituted in relation to human development. I aim to build knowledge about suffering and its origins in primordial maternal dimensions of existence that emerge in the narratives as a primary domain of moral experience for seriously ill elders. I wish also to help assure that such knowledge may be utilized to guide ethical action in advancing the goals of preventing and relieving suffering and improving systems of care for older adults. Thus, my project is animated not only by theoretical goals, but by practical goals that have important implications for creative engagement and action: the cultivation of practical wisdom as a moral response to the suffering of life-world existence, and the building up of ethics in community as lived social practice.

Within this overarching framework and through my research, I have heightened my sensitivity and attunement to lived experiences of suffering, as well as pain— especially chronic, intolerable, and intractable pain that may lead to suffering or is itself a type of embodied suffering. I have observed first-hand the varying health, social, and cultural contexts in which pain and suffering are often found, such as in situations of loss, trauma, distress, or chronic illness burden. I have also deepened my appreciation for the depth of complexity in experiences of pain and suffering, recognizing that in certain situations, pain and suffering may be present at once and entangled in ways that demand better understanding. In other situations, suffering exists in the absence of pain, and pain in the absence of suffering. The implications of my unfolding project in these contexts are social, and relevant to processes for improving not only social care provision, but the care environment and concomitant long-term services and supports for vulnerable elders with chronic or serious illness.

While much has been written in the medical literature about both pain and suffering, primarily within the dominant biomedical paradigm, my research examines pain and suffering through the lens of phenomenology (Husserl, 1913/1982, 1913/1989), building on notions of human personhood in the work of

Eric J. Cassell (1982, 2004) and others writing in the medical humanities and social sciences (Browning, 2004; Frank, 1978, 1995, 2001; Frankl, 1984; Kleinman, 1988, 2012; Miller, 2004; Sulmasy, 2002), and embedded within a larger social ecology of humanistic care and concern in which social work, psychology, nursing, and the other helping professions participate. Within this social ecology of care and concern about suffering elders, I engage in examining the meanings of elders' pain and suffering experiences, in light of social and "*I-Thou*" relational dimensions of existence (Buber, 1958/2000; Levinas, 1969; Schütz, 1967). In examining these meanings, I explore the possibility for human development, agency, spiritual flourishing, and attainment of well-being among elders journeying through narratives of illness, recovery and resilience, and transcending the porous boundaries of illness experience itself.

I have undertaken focused research on these questions. In this book, I share the major findings from my study of suffering among seriously ill older adults ("main study"), as presented primarily in narrative form, and sketch the beginning contours of a phenomenology of suffering, Maternal Affordances and Maternal-Relational Ethics. I also draw upon findings from my more recent study of pain, suffering, and decision making in follow up to the main study ("follow-up study"). The original research questions for both the main and follow-up studies emerged from my review of the gaps in the literature on pain, suffering and end-of-life decision making, my policy practice knowledge as a non-clinical practitioner, and preliminary findings of my pilot oral history project in which I explored suffering and illness burden in the life course of a frail elderly woman. I have taken multiple steps to protect the anonymity of the study participants whom I reference individually by alias names in the chapter narratives that follow, or simply as "persons," whether they resided or received care in hospital or nursing facilities. For the purposes of fully protecting study participants' anonymity, certain information is not disclosed in the narratives such as specific geographic locations, names of facilities, or places of origin. But before we turn to the narratives themselves, I must first introduce my readers to the origins and development of my project and journey, and describe the processes that I continue to chart and navigate as I write these chapters.

In all of my research engagements, I have been deliberate in bracketing my theoretical and scientific knowledge, or holding it in suspension striving for an open and impartial approach in encountering experience and analyzing data, answering my research questions, and evaluating the limitations of my research. For the social scientist as an interpreter of experience, the reflexive process is an ongoing one of constant mindfulness that is part of the larger research endeavor. The trustworthiness of my research studies has been and is enhanced by my accounting fully for my role and responsibility in the field of scientific inquiry. As part of this accounting, in utilizing phenomenological methods, I explain how I as researcher may turn to my own lived experience as a source of examples of the phenomena under study that may be imaginatively varied in eidetic analysis, and my empathic access and responses to others that may also be part of the field of experience (Wertz, 2010).

I retain a sense of surprise, as well as humility, that the major findings in my main study—a Maternal Ground and Maternal Affordances in experiences of pain and suffering in serious illness and at the end of life—were not part of my research questions, but emerged in open-ended interviews with the study participants. This element of surprise in my research findings speaks to the merits of a fresh examination of suffering experience, unimpeded by prior theories or constructs. Even in light of this freshness and impartiality that I have striven to bring to the study of suffering, however, the protocols and practices accepted in the community of qualitative researchers call for individual acknowledgment of the sensitizing experiences that framed my interests in these experiences, and deepened my capacity for empathy with those who are living through suffering. In a spirit of authenticity, it would be disingenuous not to acknowledge that all my life experiences have become a part of my temporal individuated consciousness. While I aim to bracket scientific knowledge, theoretical perspectives, and even my own experiences, my developed consciousness and foreground structure can never be expunged or completely suspended in the research process, and I remain always in a moral position of non-neutrality in that I have committed myself to a certain scientific project and my valuing of that project, especially as it concerns my orientation to the *other*. For these reasons, readers may wish to understand how I have arrived at this point in my journey, how I came to define my study focus and devote myself to this research project, and how my experiences have shaped my perspectives and my capacities for empathic access to suffering persons.

My encounter with suffering in the research investigations I have conducted at care facilities is not the first time I have been a witness to suffering, or exposed to trauma. The home has been a horizon of significance in my life experiences, beginning with my earliest years. My early childhood was a very sheltered one, in part because of the unexpected death of my father, *John V.*, when I was six weeks old. But within the warmth of the home I shared with my mother, my brother *Kevin*, and my Irish-born maternal grandparents who came to help take care of us, I enjoyed very rich experiences. There were always lively conversations at the dinner table among family members, visitors, and my mother's colleagues and friends, and the house was full of things to read and immerse myself in, from my mother's and father's cherished books on Freud and Jung, to the poetry of Henry Wadsworth Longfellow. I also spent endless, blissful hours playing outside in my yard amidst the big oak trees, the yellow forsythia, and purple hydrangea, and planting tall red salvia in the flower beds of the front garden, and I loved riding my bike across the sprawling green lawn.

I had the pleasure of spending much time and remaining close to my grandmother *Bridie*, as she was called in America, until her death in my early adulthood. She faithfully attended to my needs and my brother's, allowing my mother to earn a living and a doctorate in social work. I knew my grandmother intimately; she taught me how to read and spell, do arithmetic, and recite poetry and prayers to the Blessed Mother. Her stalwart strength in the face of adversity, her passion for learning, and her love and care for my brother and me, as well as for all little children, were a cultural legacy of her Irish upbringing.

During the time my grandparents lived with my family, my grandfather "*Di-da*," as I called him, developed diabetes and lost both of his legs. He was wheelchair-bound, and I remember sitting with him in the yard on summer days. I would find his eyeglasses for him, and bring him the sweet grape juice he loved to drink despite his illness. In her nineties, my grandmother spent her last years in a nursing facility following several strokes, alert until the end of her life despite these assaults. I would visit her often, and when I was not able to see her in person, I would talk to her every day on the phone. She was always so lonely and forlorn in the home; I can visualize her still sitting in the wheelchair by the phone waiting for a call or visit, much as I remember her gaze when she had stood at the door and watched me get on the bus for school many years earlier. She died about six weeks before my first child was born, and I was honored to name my daughter *Breda* in her memory.

Twenty-five years later I would live through a somewhat parallel experience with my mother, who suffered a hip fracture following a very painful bout of shingles, and later a pelvic fracture. Although she recovered from the hip fracture in terms of restored functioning, she never fully regained her strength and robustness. When she was no longer able to remain engaged in her work life due to her increasing frailty, she let go of it with deep reluctance, and mourned its loss. She eventually faced giving up her own home when she could no longer live independently. She came to live with my family, and took some comfort in the companionship and loving care she received. But she continued to yearn to return to work, to share conversations again with colleagues in the hallowed halls of the university where she had been a professor of social work, and later dean, for nearly 50 years. When she fell in our home and fractured her pelvis a few weeks before she died, it was her excruciating pain that I recall most vividly. She found no relief or refuge from her suffering and called for God to take her.

While I attest with honor to being a witness to my grandparents' traumatic illnesses, in reflecting upon their experiences I am not sure I comprehended the full meaning and significance of their suffering as they lived through it. When I returned to the university to begin my dissertation in 2005, well before my mother became ill, my research interests initially focused on health care decision making, but I had not yet appreciated the complex relationship of pain and suffering to decision making. As I expanded my knowledge and sensitivity through an oral history project I had the honor of doing with my mother as she lived through her traumatic experience of coping with the shingles, as well as in my ongoing research, I began to focus my interests more specifically on suffering and decision making in serious illness.

At the outset, I believe that I may have approached the study of lived experiences of pain and suffering in part as an outsider, drawing heavily on my early career education, training, and experience in health law and regulation. Not until I had immersed myself in the study of phenomenology did I really begin separating myself from these early framings as external norms, and instead begin to see the world from within a relational stance in its unvarnished complexity, ambiguity, and diversity through access to the first-person experiences and voices of suffering persons themselves and the development of human consciousness disclosed in these experiences. In a temporal moment of revelation and awe during these early phenomenology studies that continues to hold and nourish me, I made a commitment to the faithful understanding of lived experiences of pain and suffering, which I shall call my project. Of intense interest to me are the meanings that pain and suffering have for the *other*—not only the family members I have loved and have lost, but the anonymous *other* living in the nursing facility, in the hospital, or in the community, on behalf of whose dignity we labor.

I encountered Angelique for the first time in my visits to a care facility where she resided, sitting patiently in her wheelchair waiting for an elevator in the company of several other residents of the facility and the staff members assisting them. I was struck by her elegance, her upright posture in the wheelchair, her impeccable grooming, carefully braided silver hair, and brightly colored shoes. But I also observed a certain rigidity in her demeanor, and what I discerned at the time seemed to be an absence of facial expression. I immediately apprehended in her presentation a sense of pride and self-respect, even as she remained confined to her wheelchair. I wondered nevertheless whether she was in any discomfort and whether her rigidity reflected a kind of stoic response to some type of pain. I experienced a more global response to what I beheld in that environment, namely, that this was not an uncommon vignette in care facility life—frail elderly residents in wheelchairs, bracing themselves with pregnant pause for the slow march of time.

Not long after that initial encounter at the elevator, I visited Angelique in her room to introduce myself as a researcher. I invited her to participate in my study, and she agreed to speak with me as a study participant. As we completed the informed consent process, Angelique painstakingly signed the forms, drawing upon weakened bodily resources that chronic disease had depleted. In subsequent visits, I would make my way to Angelique's floor and to her room, where I would find her sitting serenely in her wheelchair. During one of my early interviews with Angelique, the care facility staff on the floor advised me that she had recently been moved into the hospice program. The staff expressed concern that Angelique did not understand this change in her goals of care, and it might cause her distress.

Over a period of six months conducting my research at the care facility, I got to know Angelique, or rather, Angelique revealed herself to me in ways that I did not anticipate. The rigid demeanor I had first observed belied a much richer tapestry of experience that Angelique described in her interviews with me, spanning her early childhood to the present. While she was English-speaking, the descriptions of her experiences were embedded in a distinctive dialect and in idiomatic expressions imbued with their own meaning.

In an interview with Angelique's social worker, I learned that Angelique was perceived as a robust advocate for her own needs among the staff at the care facility. Yet, contrary to this perception by staff, Angelique described her own feelings of not being a full participant in her care planning, especially in the decision to be admitted to hospice. This tension between her own voice and the lens of institutional processes would remain prominent in Angelique's experiences. As a frail elderly woman with multiple chronic conditions, Angelique lived with bodily pain every day. I came to understand through our conversations the multiple meanings her pain had for her, and how her pain experiences were related to dimensions of suffering she lived through in the nursing facility and at earlier times in her life history.

The individual structure of Angelique's suffering experience is based on in-depth reflective analyses. I also provide a more general understanding of the experience of suffering in serious illness based upon Angelique's and several other elders' accounts. My findings include an analysis of individual examples of the phenomenon as it appeared, followed by the more general knowledge that the study generated. These findings are "structural" in nature both at the individual and general levels, in that they disclose the complex web of relationships among the constituents of Angelique's experiences. While each constituent in the individual structure of Angelique's life-world experience is a self-contained unit with fluid boundaries that has both its own constitutive parts and an open exchange with the environment in which it is situated, the constituent relates to other constituents in a formal and ordered way, and neither the constituent nor its parts can be reduced to the ground upon which they rest. All constituents form one unified individual structure. The Maternal is the independent ground from which other constituents arise and develop, and therefore, may be described as founding in Angelique's suffering experience. In the absence of the Maternal Ground, the structure of suffering would collapse.

In Angelique's individual structure of suffering, the Maternal dimensions of existence are the ground upon which agency, sociality, and spirituality develop over Angelique's life course. In the structure of suffering, the Maternal ground is therefore the first temporal moment of experience. Angelique's transition to the care facility in a middle moment in her life course thrusts her from the well-being of her home—the anchor of her family, spiritual and religious life—into a vortex of bodily and emotional pain. Loss of Maternal foundations, especially as embodied in Angelique's supportive home surroundings, and other pervasive threats to her temporal horizons constitute core meanings of suffering for her in her end-of-life illness. Through the narrative, I use "Maternal Foundations" to describe the constituents of the structure which the Maternal founds that are part of the unified whole. I do not mean the original "Maternal Ground" itself which is independent and founding.

Angelique experiences loss in multiple dimensions: the denial of embodied care that satisfies human needs and relieves the burdens of illness; dislocation from the home and immersion in an alienating, unwelcoming realm; removal from the intimate bonds of her family, caregivers and community; a lack of support and communication with caregivers appropriate to the trauma of dislocation; and distancing from full participation in patient decision making. Angelique's feelings of marginalization in the process of making decisions about her care weaken her perceptions of self-efficacy, diminish her personal agency, and heighten her suffering. Angelique's phenomenal lived, expressive, and weeping body, and shrunken spatiality and temporal relations, both with herself and others, disclose the full affective dimensions of Angelique's suffering experiences.

In the third temporal moment, Angelique's teleological desire—a need to find meaning and closure at the end of life, especially as they relate to suffering—and intentional, agentic, life-affirming movement are directed toward self-actualizing, resilience in the face of threats and assaults on dignity, and spiritual growth and well-being. Patient decision making is a complex self- and social-developmental process, an expression of agency and palliative response to suffering that helps Angelique cope with suffering as she draws upon spiritual reserves and personal resources in living with life-threatening illness. At the end of life, Angelique journeys toward her place of origin in a Maternal homecoming, in which she struggles to emerge from varying liminal states with a reconstituted self.

Although the narrative account of Angelique's life-history that I share in this book is a richly descriptive one, in both the main and follow-up studies, I also draw upon narratives of other frail elderly study participants residing in care facilities who have lived through experiences of pain and/or suffering. Both the variations in these experiences, as well as their essential dimensions, are important to understand and honor. I attempt to give a faithful portrait of the depth and complexity of these experiences in the chapters that follow.

The goal of this particular book is neither an in-depth explication of research methods, nor a treatise in philosophy. Rather, the focus is narrowly concerned with describing and understanding suffering experience and the process of how suffering is constituted. This is a narrative project that remains unfinished in the sense that it is always unfolding—directed toward the telos of an authentic life in the face of suffering, but eluding certainty. In the opening chapter, I describe the suitability of qualitative inquiry to my research interests. In particular, I aim to convey the power of phenomenological methods—the rigorous phenomenological procedures adhered to in the analysis of my data—to access persons' everyday and often invisible experiences of suffering. I also place phenomenology in its historical contexts in relationship to the disciplines of philosophy and psychology, and explore the fruitfulness of these relationships to understanding the experience of human suffering within the scope of the project. I describe elder suffering, among its others dimensions, in epistemological, ontological, symbolic and ethical terms, and identify the constituents of the Maternal Ground disclosed in my research as essential to the structure of suffering, its founding relationship to elders' development at the end of life in locating freedom and finding hope, and to the design of Maternal environments and systems of care.

Drawing upon the salient features of phenomenology in its fidelity to the subject and lived experience, its focus on intentionality, intersubjectivity, and the primacy of the ethical relation to the other, my goals in the chapters that follow are to describe elder suffering as it is witnessed by neighbors, in communities, and across nations. In Chapters 2 through 4, I present the narrative account of the life of Angelique in its three temporal moments, primarily a genetic phenomenological analysis describing how Angelique's experiences are constituted from their very beginning or ground. I start with Angelique's descriptions in the present, in her own idiom and dialect, and trace them back to a primordial Maternal experience in her origins. In addition to Angelique, I develop the narratives of several older women and men in Chapters 5 through 7, focusing on individual experiences of suffering and care-seeking experiences, as well as cultural and community care perspectives. I highlight a general structure of suffering that I have identified in my research studies and as central to such structure, the prominence of Maternal dimensions of existence that are a primary domain of moral experience for suffering elders. Through these narrative accounts, I attempt to sketch a tentative and beginning phenomenology for understanding the fabric of this moral experience in serious illness and suffering, and the development of moral consciousness, obligation, and agency in relation to meaningful others and the social world. Finally, in Chapter 8, I discuss the general structure of suffering in the narratives in more depth, and comment on the practical implications of the recovered social worlds of suffering elders for policy, interdisciplinary practice and research, as well as for bioethical inquiry. The intended audience for this book includes scholars who may be interested in phenomenology as a philosophy and research method, educators, and practitioners—social workers, psychologists, nurses, physicians, chaplains, and ethicists who are working with seriously ill persons and their family members, and law practitioners counseling older adults, their family members, and health providers.

1 The Dialectics of Suffering and Maternal Care-Seeking in Serious Illness

The famous painting from Picasso's Blue Period, *The Old Guitarist*, captures so effectively both elder suffering and the rising of hope in the midst of suffering. At the center of the painting is the guitar and its promise of music, and the suggestion that this promise seems to anchor the blind, melancholic old man whose grip on life is tenuous. The full aesthetic dimensionalities of Picasso's image give access to a unified temporal moment of suffering in tension with hope, as well as the ambiguity inherent in this moment.

The problem of suffering among older adults, as depicted in Picasso's *The Old Guitarist*, has not garnered sufficient attention and is understudied. The nature of the problem is complex, spanning social, ecological, and public health domains, and involving concerns about perception, epistemology as well as ontology, provision and ethics of care, and moral obligation and agency. The epistemological aspects of suffering may be framed in terms of accessing the suffering of the other. The problem of care presents challenges in how we respond to the suffering other. In this inquiry, I seek to understand the nature of suffering—widely viewed as situated within an existing biomedical paradigm—its origins, horizons, contexts, manifestations, and temporal movement as understood both within the scientific community and among non-scientists. The dominant biomedical paradigm, that gives primacy to curative and pharmacologic approaches to treatment, is now being called into question as part of a shift in how suffering is conceptualized. Discrepant evidence about experience of suffering and care responses to suffering that motivate recovery and resilience are prompting a move away from a purely medical perspective to a reframing of suffering as part of our human development over the life course. These reframings tease out the tension between the common sense understanding of health as an achievement of natural science and technical rationality, and the lived experience of health as an achievement of ethics grounded in social practices. They invite reflection on the gap between concrete reality, the things themselves that phenomenology allows access to, and the paradigms of science upon which conventional notions about health and health systems have been constructed. Such paradigm shifts are patterns that have been formally recognized by scholars such as Thomas Kuhn (1962), who have illuminated the role of social contexts in scientific revolutions. The emerging paradigm is fundamentally social and relational, not only helping remove barriers to understanding, but promoting more empathic access to diverse meanings in ethical encounter with suffering persons and more effective responses to such suffering in essentially and relationally constitutive human ways.

Framings of Pain and Suffering: Conceptual Swamp

A "conceptual swamp" in the medical and medical humanities literature has muddied understanding of suffering as phenomenologically distinct from pain (Morrissey, 2011a, p.18), a subject that will be elaborated on throughout the chapters of this book. Eric J. Cassell's (1982, 1999, 2004) description of suffering as an experience that threatens the intactness of the person and personhood is often cited as the authoritative scholarship on the subject of suffering. In his work on suffering, Cassell developed a topology of the person and personhood that he described as being broader than the concept of self, positing that there are parts of the person that are not part of the self, may be known by others, but not by me. His conceptualization takes account of the bodily, social, cultural, emotional, instrumental, political, relational, historical, familial, and transcendent dimensions of personhood. Cassell also describes processes that involve personal interpretation of illness experiences and symptoms, and the assignment of meanings to such experiences. However, Cassell remains firmly committed to the personal, private and individual nature of suffering. While Cassell's conceptualization has informed the scholarly dialogue on person-centered care and laid an important foundation for future scholarly inquiry, it does not sufficiently account for the social constitution of suffering (Morrissey, 2011b). Pain is defined somewhat more narrowly in the scientific literature as a sensory and emotional experience that involves bodily tissues, or actual or potential tissue damage (International Association for the Study of Pain [IASP], 2011), yet like suffering in some sense involves annihilation of self and world. These framings of pain and suffering share considerable overlap, and are often blurred. Generally, there is a growing and robust body of science on pain, and a newly emerging focus on developing a national pain agenda as the result of the 2011 Institute of Medicine (IOM) blueprint report on pain prevalence and pain disparities in the United States (IOM, 2011). In particular, the problem of chronic pain, its etiology, social determinants, and the design of effective approaches to its treatment are posing new challenges for researchers and practitioners (Atlas & Skinner, 2010; Gatchel, McGeary, McGeary, & Lippe, 2014; Institute of Medicine, 2011; Jensen & Turk, 2014). However, the study of suffering remains a neglected area of scientific inquiry. Through the narrative accounts in this book, a sharpened focus is brought to bear on descriptions and definitions that blur understanding of the phenomenality of pain and suffering as distinct experiences, and as part of that process, prevailing views and their underpinnings are called into question. For example, it is suggested that pain is an experience that may not always involve actual or potential tissue damage, as set forth in the IASP definition.

Narrative is a method that has been used extensively by scholars such as Arthur Frank (1995), Arthur Kleinman (1988), Kathy Charmaz (1983; 1997; 1999), Mark Freeman (2008a, 2008b), Ruthellen Josselson (Josselson, 2013; Wertz et al.,

2011), as well as others (Black, 2006; Burlea, 2009; De Beauvoir, 1965; Good, 1994), in aiming to capture the voice and agency of the suffering other and the ethical relation to the other in lived experiences of illness, aging and dementia (Morrissey, 2014a, 2014c). The literature suggests that suffering may be concerned with experiences of loss and distress, and with a search for meaning (Altilio, 2004; Black, 2006; Byock, 1996; Charmaz, 1983, 1997, 1999; Ferrel & Coyle, 2008; Frankl, 1984). Narrative method is part of the shift away from explanatory approaches to the scientific investigation of suffering rooted in the current dominant biomedical models of disease diagnosis and treatment, and toward relational models of assessment, intervention and decision making that restore ethics as a central ground of humanistic understanding in the interdisciplinary study of social development and taken-for-granted experiences of suffering in everyday life (Miller, 2004; Morrissey & Jennings, 2006; Morrissey, 2011a, 2011b). Drawing on Virginia Woolf's "A Room of One's Own" (1957), it is asserted that the proper locus of writing, and in the present context narrative writing, is—"not in re-living or re-telling, but in more fully embodying the presence of reality—the moment which transcends temporality" and "that which is perpetually in a state of flux" (Morrissey, 1979, p. 4–5). In the last pages of "A Room of One's Own," Woolf describes the stream of experience that is existence as "the common life which is the real life and not… the little separate lives which we live as individuals" (p. 114).

The salient dimensions of suffering that have been prominent in my research findings and inform the suffering narratives of older adults are its excruciating immediacy, and unbounded or boundless and indeterminate qualities, and its presence to the experiencing person as such. While all things may be said to be situated against a horizon of indeterminacy, it is suggested that the human encounter with these essential dimensions of suffering arises in the context of socially and culturally constituted losses of Maternal Foundations. It is the immediate, unbounded and indeterminate dimensionalities of suffering, embedded dialectically within conditions of human finitude, temporality, and ambiguity that creates the feeling that there is no refuge from it. My research findings also suggest that these qualities of suffering cannot be easily translated into concepts and language, and may be fully accessible only at pre-conceptual and pre-theoretical levels of experience, or through non-linguistic forms of expression in art, and music and poetry. Based on these tentative findings, suffering appears as qualitatively different from more finite experiences of illness and non-chronic pain. For these reasons, I have sought descriptions of suffering that will help to deepen our understanding of it, especially in light of its elusive nature. In the last chapter of the book, I attempt to integrate all the findings as presented in the narratives and provide a fuller explication of a proposed tentative general structure of suffering that shows its essential constituents as suffering, the *thing itself*. We know and may say then with certainty that suffering exists empirically, yet we continue to be faced with uncertainty about its *whatness* and how it is constituted. Suffering therefore escapes definition as a concrete problem, and cannot be cured through technical and material interventions or solutions, even if it can at times be relieved.

Maternal Dimensions of Existence as Primary Domain of Moral Experience

Perhaps no work of art in our lifetime so powerfully and profoundly conveys the multiple intersecting realities and meanings of suffering and its associated lost Maternal Foundations, especially in the context of communities, as Picasso's *Guernica*. Picasso depicts horrific violence and death amidst a community of humans and animals—a dying horse, a dying soldier, and a weeping, bereft mother with head swung back holding her dead baby. As in the painting of the old man and his guitar, Picasso evokes hope in the symbol of a small flower in the midst of a scorched landscape of death and dismemberment. The aesthetic achievements of Picasso and other great artists enrich our capacity to see what is not immediately evident or visible, but may be hidden and invisible. This is the archeological task of phenomenology in the present project—recovering and making visible the social worlds of suffering elders.

Toward a Phenomenology of the Maternal

In the chapters that follow, I interrogate the Maternal as it has appeared in my research studies in the context of suffering—*the Maternal*, as the "thing itself" or concrete reality (which I shall reference as "the Maternal"), as explicated by philosopher Edmund Husserl in his description of the phenomenological turn (Husserl, 1901/1970; Wertz, 2010) or by French phenomenologist Gabriel Marcel (1949) in his attention to concrete being as grasped through secondary reflection, and its appearance in the temporal horizons of suffering experience as an independent ground of relationality and interembodiment: temporality, spatiality, and the home; perception and intersubjectivity; and agency and spirituality. I aim in this inquiry to begin tracing the contours of a phenomenology of the Maternal in its temporal and dialectical movements and horizonal entanglements with suffering experience – from the origin and genetic constitution of suffering to the re-constitution of consciousness in the affordances of the Maternal. This is a genetic phenomenological analysis, focused on locating the beginnings and contexts of suffering. My goal is to uncover layers of experience and meaning, using the descriptive and reflective analysis methods of phenomenology, that may not be visible in ordinary everyday lives, or which may not be amenable to description or verbal expression using the language of "pain" or "suffering." These methods involve the researcher's engagement of the person being interviewed in a face-to-face encounter and bodily rapport, skills of focused attention, sensitive listening and attunement, and immersion in the qualitative data collected (Wertz, 2005; Churchill, 2010; Josselson, 2013). Employing this qualitative approach to inquiry, which has been described as "retrieval" or "depth phenomenology" (Churchill, 2010, p. 86), opens up access to meanings that may be hidden, but revelatory in helping to demystify suffering experience.

The meanings of the Maternal that I have accessed in the main and follow-up studies are multiple, and include the constituents of empathy, receptivity, Maternal holding and cradling, relational intimacy and generosity, unconditional loving care, and well-being and generativity in a welcoming home. I make a clear distinction between the Maternal as a general experience, and what is more commonly described as "mothering," meaning the parenting of a child by a biological mother or mother surrogate, although this is not excluded from the general. I draw upon a broader concept of the Maternal that describes a certain given or condition of possibility in lived-through ordinary experiences of women, as well as men, who have never been biological mothers, surrogates, or parents. This concept of the Maternal builds on earlier work on the mother–child relationship defined in the literature on attachment (Bowlby, 1957, 1958, 1960, 1965, 1989; Bretherton, 1992), psychoanalysis (Freud, 1948, 1952, 1954, 1965), and developmental psychology (Winnicott, 1965; DeRobertis, 2010). However, it expands this earlier work in framing the Maternal as "pre-given" or a condition of possibility in the lived world not confined to the sphere of influence of the mother figure alone, or to the dyadic relationship, but as belonging to a larger social ecology. Maternal dimensions of existence may be located in social networks (Takahashi, 2005), and in non-human things such as the ground we walk on that supports us, the food we eat that nurtures us, or music that holds us, soothes us, and gives us comfort. I attempt to expand consciousness of the Maternal as a ground of the intentional structure of suffering and how it manifests itself in Maternal care-seeking behavior. More generally, the structure of the Maternal as I have articulated it forms a ground for an elder's founding subject-world intentional connection, as situated against changing horizons and contexts, and in the process of recovering the full life of consciousness and engagement with the world. For the older adults in the chapter narratives, experience of the Maternal—recollected and re-enacted in later life—is thematized in the anchoring presence of the Maternal Ground. In its independence from suffering experience, the Maternal is also the ground of human dignity and irreducible personhood—from womb to worlding at birth, in the processes of becoming from birth to death, and in reflective moral action and creative freedom (Marcel, 1949, 1964).

Maternal Ground and Maternal Affordances

The concept of ground as founding is by no means a new one. It figured prominently in Husserl's description of origins and horizons (Husserl, 1901/1970; Stapleton, 1983), and more contemporary phenomenologists such as Gail Weiss (2008) have made it central to the understanding of identity and social change. In identifying a general structure of suffering to which the Maternal is essential, I identify the Maternal as its own *eidos* of significance—independent from suffering, but founding suffering. The Maternal is a founding first, and borrowing from Gabriel Marcel (1949), a "presence," (p. 111), "plenitude" (p. 86), or "disposability" (p. 69). Suffering is a falling away from this fullness of being—a condition of our "ontological deficiency" (Marcel, 1949, p. 174). In this sense of suffering, it has tragic dimensions, understood so well by many of the philosophers—Marcel, as well as Hegel, who had a special interest in Sophocles' *Antigone*, the Greek tragedy, and its meanings (Roche, 2005; Westphal, 1998).

I have adopted the term "Maternal Affordances" to more fully describe the Maternal Ground and, in keeping with the seminal work of James Gibson (1979), the possibilities that the Maternal Ground makes available to the other. I describe the Maternal as an absolute availability. According to McGrenere and Ho (2000), Gibson's concept of an affordance is "an action possibility available in the environment to an individual, independent of the individual's ability to perceive this possibility" (p. 179). This is important to our understanding of Maternal Affordances as in some instances, possibilities are perceived by suffering persons and in others they are not, but may still be acted upon.

The Scope and Magnitude of Suffering

Suffering among individual older adults must be understood in the context of both its scope and magnitude among older adults writ large, from data on pain prevalence and the relationship of pain to chronic illness and multimorbidity (Morrissey, Viola, & Shi, 2014), to increasing frailty and dependency (Lunney, Lynn, & Hogan, 2002), to the larger health system issues of fragmentation and the absence of comprehensive policy in long-term care. This environment of global or social suffering (Kleinman & Kleinman, 1997) among elders has created urgency as well as opportunity for changes in care paradigms for older adults. Palliative care and the palliative ethic of care (Fins, 2006) have emerged as a prominent evidence-based paradigm that holds promise for offering elders optimal care at all stages of the illness trajectory, from early chronic illness through the end of life. Its primary goals are identification of patients with unmet care needs using targeting criteria such as dementia, frailty and functional decline; prevention and relief of pain and suffering through pain and symptom management; patient, family and caregiver support; and provision of practical and social supports (Center to Advance Palliative Care, 2014; Gomez-Baptiste, Martinez-Munoz, Blay, Espinosa, Contel, & Ledesma, 2012; National Consensus Project, 2013). Supporting older adults in their homes as long as possible is critically important to preventing dependency and avoiding institutionalization, as well as the detrimental consequences associated with traumatic care transitions.

Epistemological and Ontological Aspects of Suffering

Understanding the problem of knowledge in elder care—how we know the suffering of the elder other and how we access the elder's experience of suffering—will allow the design of appropriate palliative care services to most effectively meet the needs of elders. I would define this knowledge problem broadly as: "How do we know the suffering of the elder other, and how do we access the elder's experience of suffering?" The conventional view for many decades has deemed suffering to be wholly personal, private, and inaccessible (Cassell, 1982, 2004), and "self" and "other" as separate from the very beginning, although this view or perspective is corrigible or subject to correction. While it is well-established that persons undergo originary experiences available only to themselves, there is ample evidence, especially through studies in phenomenology (Wertz 1985, 2005; Churchill, 2010), indicating that we can know and gain access to the other in sufficient ways to establish a ground for empathy and care. Phenomenological methods show that the originarily given experience of the subject is not given to any other person as originary experience. In other words, the second person can never stand in the same shoes of the subject, or directly occupy the consciousness, experiences, and worldview of the unique individual subject. However, in the context of illness and suffering and the subject-other relationship, this does not mean, in wholesale terms or as a matter of universal principle, that the person's suffering experiences are never accessible by any other person in any form. The person's suffering experience may be accessed by the other, but not in the very same way as it is given to or experienced by the subject alone in his or her own temporal stream of consciousness (Morrissey & Barber, 2014). For example, Morrissey and Barber (2014) have explained that the person who is suffering is living through his or her suffering as embodied, or through the lived body, as a body-subject in a world that is present to others. The person's lived body is also a body in the world available to others, and like "my" body. This access to the psychological subject in the experience of the face-to-face encounter and through an intersubjective bodily relation has been described by Scott Churchill (2010) as the "second person perspective" or "awareness" (p. 84). According to Husserl (1989), however, this knowledge of suffering through experience would never be complete and adequate because it is never given originally to me. But as experience *qua* experience, it is meaningful not only for epistemic reasons, but because it is evidential—constitutive evidence of the presence of suffering in the world—and therefore has ontological significance.

In this context of accessing the suffering other, I turn to philosopher Henry Bugbee (1958) who in *Inward Morning* describes the concreteness of experience and the certainty that belongs to all experience for those who choose to immerse themselves in the lived world of experience. I appeal to this concreteness and certainty of experience in describing suffering as absolute, unable to be denied, and so prominent in existence that it stands out visibly and boldly in the tapestry of all existence and experiences. The perception of suffering in this sense— suffering that is made significant by our essential humanity, vulnerability, and finitude—is not problematic. I see it and recognize it when it appears before me, although I can never have complete knowledge of its absoluteness. Suffering manifests itself in the world as a determinacy of indeterminacy: we are certain of its presence and terrible reality, yet its reality consists in its essential indeterminacy, inconsistency, impenetrability, and mystery. Because of these qualities, suffering can never be justified or fully accounted for through rational understanding, but we can describe it as it appears to us and through description try to deepen our understanding of it.

A focus on the elder other, the "priority of the other" as psychologist Mark Freeman has written about (Freeman, 2013), and the elder as *other*—the thematized experience of the elder as the *other* who makes a moral claim on us, need to be informed most importantly by the first person perspective of elders themselves, that is, their own descriptions of their life histories and lived experiences of suffering. These first person perspectives and voices of elders, and the systematic reflections on them in the process of scientific inquiry that disclose the essential constituents of suffering experience—in other words, the "engines" of the experience without which the experience would not occur—deepen our understanding of elders' meanings and expressions. We also need to incorporate the "second person" (Churchill, 2010, p. 84) perspective of elders' experiences from the standpoint and positionality of caregivers—both family and professional—as we know that elder care presents significant challenges for caregivers (Gonzalez Sanders & Fortinsky, 2012; Reinhard, Levine, & Samis, 2012; Reinhard, Levine, & Samis, 2014). There is a sense in which caregiving is not only an interpersonal lens, but an ecological systems perspective. This perspective is well-established in social work practice with children and families (Webb, 2011) and must inform our understanding of elder experience. This continuum of perspectives of experiences of elder suffering—from the personal to the interpersonal, interprofessional, and ecological—is integral to the more global contexts in which elders are situated.

Lastly, we need to amplify and magnify our focus on the ethical encounter with the elder as other, the intersubjective nexus between elder and caregiver that is the locus of relationality, empathy, care, communication, and palliation of suffering. The ethical encounter with the elder other also extends to the researcher who enters into a covenantal commitment to the elder from the moment of first encounter. This commitment involves not only respecting the dignity, privacy, and personal boundaries of the person, but even beyond these basic relational affirmations, creating a sacred space that is shared with the elder in recognition of the mutual vulnerability and limitations of finite human beings, and in a willingness to surrender positions of authority (Benjamin, 2004; Rogers, 1961). Let there be no question that this commitment is a moral position, and a rejection of the logical positivistic view of value-free scientific inquiry. Psychologist Ronald B. Miller (2004) describes the claim to moral neutrality in science and clinical practice as "based on a misunderstanding of the nature of moral and ethical principles" (p. 20). The moral and ethical are fundamentally concerned with what one should do in fulfillment of one's intentionalities, and the moral choices and evaluations one makes in pursuit of the good, a good life, and human flourishing, in keeping with Aristotle's conception of *eudaimonia*. John Drummond (2002) argues that a phenomenological, neo-Aristotelian ethics involves a teleological, eudaimonsitic and non-consequentialist notion of the good. Drummond (2002, 2008a) elaborates further on the multiple dimensions of ethics: apprehension of the moral rooted in everyday experience; norms for ethical conduct; and in the third dimension, a focus on the moral *agent* and the moral goods of agency. In the chapter narratives that follow, there is a central focus on this third dimension of ethics—moral agency.

Humanistic psychologist Carl Rogers (1961) articulated the notion of valuing the other, and the other's "unconditional self-worth" (p.34)," as fundamental to engaging a humanistic attitude in relationship with the other. The demand for unconditional valuing described by Rogers stems from the inalienable human dignity, irreducible personhood and otherness of each person that delimits the relationship with the other, and grounds respect for the other's self-actualizing process. It is in this space that communication may occur with authentic concern for the elder other as a human person who suffers as I do, whom I accept without judgment or evaluation, and with whom I may in turn be genuine and real about my feelings—what Rogers (1961) called "congruence" (p. 50). Rogers characterized this type of helping relation that integrates unconditional valuing, congruence, and empathic understanding as affording the greatest freedom and opportunity for personal growth. For the suffering elder whose Maternal care-seeking reveals a self-actualizing and agentic drive toward mature development, the Maternal Ground and its Maternal Affordances as disclosed in the suffering narratives of older adults are a faithful rendering of the infinite possibility for development and transformation—and fulfillment of a teleological moral agency—in engagement with a humanistic attitude of openness and receptivity toward the other.

The quest for knowledge and scientific investigations—essentially rational inquiries and enterprises—must make room for that which does not fit easily into paradigms of technical rationality. Otherwise, there is a risk of excluding meanings at the margin of experience, such as the uncanny and the magical described by Freud (1919), or that which may remain a mystery as Marcel (1949) reminded us. Husserl defined reason broadly to include all position-taking—theoretical, axiological, and practical (Husserl, 1962; Stapleton, 1983). A grasp of elders' suffering should not be limited to theoretical reason only and its products, but should also accommodate what occurs at the level of pre-reflective, non-inferential thought as in experience of the common sense world, as well as what may exceed or transcend it (Barber, 2011). In these suffering narratives, elders' descriptions of their experiences reveal enactments—and re-enactments—of retained, passively synthesized experiences. These enactments and re-enactments occur at the pre-reflective level and implicate and engage elders' fully embodied emotional drives.

Phenomenology and Phenomenological Methods

The qualitative research methods employed in the main descriptive study of suffering among seriously ill older adults in an urban care facility setting, as well as in the follow-up study conducted at two different care facility sites, were phenomenological, adhering to phenomenological research procedures outlined by Giorgi (1970, 2009) and Wertz (1983a, 1983b, 1985, 2005, 2008, 2010; Wertz, Charmaz, McMullen, Josselson, Anderson, & McSpadden, 2011). As both a philosophy and a rigorous human science with a primary focus on human consciousness, phenomenology is well-suited to the focus of this project. Developed as a method for qualitative inquiry in psychology by Amedeo Giorgi, phenomenology is now used more broadly in disciplines such as social work, sociology and nursing to investigate lived experiences, and is situated in a larger post-modern movement of "institutionalization" of qualitative research in the human sciences (Wertz, 2014 , p. 12).

Phenomenological research has been a fruitful approach in the main and follow-up studies from which the narrative data for this book have been drawn because it has provided the analytic power and conceptual grasp to access and explore the experiences and meanings of frail elderly (and some young-old) persons, from their own subjective perspectives as they negotiated chronic, life-limiting, and sometimes life-threatening illness. In addressing human problems and needs, and in providing deeper access to personal and shared experiences than would be typically afforded by conventional natural science or quantitative research methods, phenomenological methods are poised to respond to the concerns and distress of persons, families, and communities that are struggling with suffering and illness burden (Morrissey, 2011b; Morrissey & Barber, 2014).

Phenomenology's strength lies in the sharp focus it brings to bear in study of the social world as a region or distinctive area of being, sometimes called a regional ontology (Wertz, 2010). This kind of study focus calls for a different methodology from those of the natural sciences. In natural science studies, in which only the scientist is viewed as an arbiter or interpreter of experience, the primary focus is the physical world and presupposed physical things as objects of research study (Morrissey & Barber, 2013). Studies that utilize these methods may yield factual and sensory data about quality of life for seriously ill elderly persons, including their objectively measurable pain and symptoms, somatic sensations, and other clinical profiles that aid in understanding an elderly person's current and changing clinical course. However, these quantitative studies and measurement tools alone do not provide the deep, empathic access to the life-worlds of frail and seriously ill elderly persons, their intentionalities, consciousness, and meanings of suffering and chronic pain in social context (Morrissey, 2011b).

Phenomenology, and a phenomenological ethics that draws on a Husserlian perspective, challenge the validity of the third-person perspective of the natural sciences and the physical world that lies at the basis of a medicalized model of health care and objective approaches to measurement of disease symptoms, diagnosis, and treatment of illness (Morrissey & Barber, 2014). Although phenomenology is sometimes viewed as antinaturalistic—that is, concerned with the social world as distinct from the natural world—it is more accurate to describe phenomenology as positively building knowledge through reflection on the structures of experience. This type of reflective knowledge complements the quantitative knowledge generated by the natural sciences, which have historically excluded the experiencing subject or perceiver from defined fields of legitimate scientific inquiry into the material, physical world.[1] Phenomenology also has relevance to critical issues in bioethics that center around the fundamentally social nature of human beings and their ecologies of health and well-being.

Edmund Husserl, viewed as the founder of phenomenology, radically altered the qualitative approach to accessing experience and data by giving a lens on the world as experienced and lived through by the intending subject, not simply the internal workings of the subject's mind (Wertz et al., 2011). The phenomenological methods he developed allow two very important methodological steps in scientific investigation: to describe experience; and to reflect on experience in order to understand the meaning of experience as meant by the subject. Husserl's methodological contributions to phenomenology, originally employed in philosophical analyses of consciousness, were adapted by Husserl himself over a period of more than 35 years to address the problems of psychology (Wertz et al., 2011). Maurice Merleau-Ponty (1962), Alfred Schütz (1967), and Emmanuel Levinas (1969), and more recently, Amedeo Giorgi (1970, 2009) and Frederick J. Wertz (2005, 2010) in psychology, and Michael Barber (2011), John Drummond (2008), and Lester Embree (1997, 2010a, 2010b) in philosophy, are among the phenomenological scholars who have advanced and modified Husserl's ideas and extended them to the full range of the humanities and social science (Morrissey, 2011b).

Husserl uses *epochés* (a word borrowed from ancient Greek generally meaning a suspension of judgment to allow for objective evaluation) or "abstentions" to accomplish these methodological steps (Wertz, 1985, p. 168; Wertz et al., 2011). The first *epoché*, the *epoché* of the natural sciences, demands a setting aside of all scientific theories, hypotheses, research, and scientific findings that pertain to the subject matter under investigation. This *epoché* gives access to what Husserl called the life-world, as experienced in the "natural attitude" in the everyday world, the world of taken-for-granted experiences, the world as it exists during the course of ordinary experience. The second *epoché*, called the *epoché* of the natural attitude, requires a "bracketing" of naive beliefs in the existence of the world and in the existence of all the things in the world. Investigation focuses instead on appearances and the meanings of those appearances as revealed by the intentionalities of the subject. In this methodological attitude, the researcher engages in reflection on the world's manner of givenness and the meanings of the full panoply of human experiences from the perspective of the experiencing subject, without passing judgment on the existence or nonexistence of what is experienced. The implications of this bracketing procedure is that there is no concern with the veridicality or non-veridicality of the subject's experiences, only with their meanings. The field of meaning may also be expanded to include the researcher's own meaning responses to the experiencing subject, without validating them. This entire process of interrogating the field of meaning, called the psychological phenomenological reduction (Wertz et al., 2011), allows the investigator to focus on the world as experienced—the world as it shows itself in experience—rather than on the independent existence of the world. This methodological attitude is a good fit for the first-person suffering and illness narratives of elderly persons discussed in this book.

There is a third transcendental *epoché* that brackets the world and puts it out of play, as Husserl (1970) described:

... a completely different sort of universal epoche is possible, namely, one which puts out of action, with one blow, the total performance running through the whole of natural world-life and through the whole network (whether concealed or open) of validities—precisely that total performance which, as the coherent "natural attitude," makes up "simple" "straightforward" ongoing life. ... An attitude is arrived at which is *above* the pregivenness of the validity above the world, ... *above* the whole manifold but synthetically unified flow in which the world has and forever attains anew its content of meaning and its ontic validity. In other words, we thus have an attitude *above* the universal conscious life (both individual-subjective and intersubjective) through which the world is "there" for those naively absorbed in onging life ... They are all put out of action in advance by the epoche, and with them the whole natural ongoing life which is directed toward the actualities of the world.

(p. 150)

Husserl (1970) goes on to explain in the *Crisis of European Sciences and Transcendental Phenomenology* that the effect of this transcendental *epoché* is to liberate oneself from the pre-givenness of the world, permitting a focus on the correlation, as he calls it, between world consciousness or transcendental subjectivity and the objective world of validities.

Moving through the performance of the various *epochés*, which involves shifts in attitude, it becomes possible to see more clearly how this type of phenomenological analysis in the Husserlian tradition may be helpful in understanding experiences of pain and suffering. Davidson and Cosgrove (2002) have explained how the "transcendental turn" is necessary to a fully developed understanding of the lived experiences of the psychological subject in the world. By performing the transcendental *epoché*, the researcher gains access to the transcendentally constituted world of consciousness, which is a world of both actively and passively synthesized or generated meanings. The individual psychological subject's immediately visible experience of suffering, for example, is embedded in a horizon of meanings and contexts that need to be uncovered through the transcendental *epoché* and transcendental reduction of phenomenological philosophy. These steps allow engagement in a genetic phenomenological analysis at the transcendental level, going back to the origins of the meanings of a phenomenon under study, to determine how it was actively and passively constituted by consciousness. According to Davidson and Cosgrove (2003), the constituting activity of transcendental subjectivity is not the activity of a single psychological subject, but involves intersubjectively constituted activity. Davidson and Cosgrove (2002) make clear that once the transcendental *epoché* is performed, it is possible to return to the lived world having recovered and made visible concealed meanings in the horizon of experience such as suffering. In summary, the four steps of the *epoché* as described by Davidson and Cosgrove are: "1) the return to the life-world from the natural attitude; 2) the phenomenological psychological reduction to the personal attitude; ... 3) securing the transcendental perspective as that from which we then 4) return to positivity to reclaim psychology as a worldly, but no longer naïve, discipline" (p. 143). Finally, transcendental subjectivity is understood to be the only pre-given in the world that is given absolutely.

In applying the transcendental turn to the study and analyses of pain and suffering experiences of frail elderly, it becomes clear that these experiences are also transcendentally constituted and involve passive syntheses, as well as active constitution of meanings. The chapter narratives provide examples of how this works. Transcendental subjectivity also helps differentiate between pain and suffering in grasping how each is constituted. The structure of suffering is distinct from pain in that it involves a movement from passively generated meanings, a condition for subjective activity, to the loss of all passivity that resides in the pre-reflective, common sense world. This means that the intentional connection between subjectivity and the objective, pre-given world of sedimented meanings is severed. This conception of suffering as arising from the decentralization of the self—a self cut off from the social world and its social moorings—is captured by David Bakan (1968) in his description of the social telos and the process of telic decentralization that threatens human flourishing.

A description of the general method of phenomenology for the purposes of the research studies and narratives in this book would not be complete without proper attention to Husserl's account of eidetic intuition, which expands conceptual comprehension of subjective experiences by faithfully articulating their essential organization and meanings. Wertz (2010) provides the following explanation of what Husserl means by "essence" as an object of knowledge:

> In his focus on "essence," Husserl revives ancient philosophical wisdom in order to address pressing scientific problems. Husserl reaffirms the view that intelligence includes the power to distinguish the essential from the accidental, and that the essential, the *eidos*, is presented objectively (Cobb Stevens, 1992). That is, the *eidos* (Plato's term [Smith, 2007]) of a subject matter is evident in the way it presents itself. Cobb-Stevens (1990, 1992, 2002) elaborates Husserl's kinship with Aristotle and his application of ancient philosophy to contemporary science. In emphasizing our grasp of objectivity unmediated by mental representations, Husserl reaffirms the primacy of seeing and intellectual insight over hypotheses, language and historical constructions. Grounded in perception and predication, in what Husserl calls intuition, knowledge takes up real situations and not mental substitutes. To see and to say that "the paper is white" is not to have a mental idea of "white" but to grasp the paper itself through its "look," the whiteness belonging to the paper (Cobb-Stevens, 1990). The paper is white. The German word *Wesen* (essence) is derived from *was* (what) and *sein* (is) (Smith, 2007). In Husserl's view, the seeing of essence provides the most fundamental knowledge of what is.
>
> (Wertz, 2010, pp. 262–263)

Phenomenological methods expand epistemological boundaries in the study of suffering through an eidetic analysis that goes beyond empirical experience and seeks to identify what is essential to experiences of suffering, such as emotions. In the main research study, as well as the follow-up study, emotions were found to play a central role in suffering because they have something to do with how persons value their experience. Eidetic analysis helps us imagine what suffering is like in terms of those aspects that we may not be able to access in a person's originary experience, because the suffering may be so extreme or remote from our own experience that we cannot see any similarities that allow us to assimilate it. For example, if we have never experienced what it is like to be so ill as to not be able to drink, to be thirsty and not be able to satiate one's thirst, to face a death of suffering from thirst and hunger because one's body can no longer assume the burden of eating and drinking, we can turn only to our imaginations to understand from a deeply human perspective what it is like as a finite human being with limited capacities to experience this type of extreme suffering.

Drawing on this explanation, both the main study and follow-up study present the question of whether the essence of lived-through experiences of suffering may be initially grasped by intuition. Intuition, as Wertz (2010) says, is an act of apprehension or perception of the givenness of an object. Eidetic analysis is a useful tool, in particular for the disclosure of suffering in lived experience, because of the inaccessibility of suffering to more traditional measures and understandings. It is clear, based upon Husserl's account of eidetic intuition, that the essence of suffering can be grasped as a phenomenon in the world presented originally to our intuition. Such a seeing necessarily involves moving through a systematic process from passively synthesized "typifications" to "exemplifications" at a higher level of generality (Wertz, 2010). From such seeing or discerning of the essence of suffering for *what* it is, not simply *that* it is, it is possible to elaborate the general structure of suffering experiences in serious illness and at the end of life that go beyond the individual experience of one subject in the world. According to Wertz (2010), through this process intuition is raised to an analytic level by employing the practice of free imaginative variation and of grasping the invariant structure of the subject matter, which would be the essence, in this case, of suffering. This notion of a general structure of lived experience must be understood as separate and distinct from an analysis of experience that focuses on intentional consciousness.

In the context of the seriously ill or frail older adult whose suffering experiences have intentional affective and motivational dimensions, eidetic intuition permits understanding of the older adult's experiences, not simply for that particular older adult in his or her subjective performances and the meanings she/he assigns to them, but at another level, as examples *qua* examples of suffering. When we employ eidetic intuition, we may find that experiences of suffering have a certain essence or core present in all instances of suffering (Wertz, 2010). The method of imaginative variation, which notes the invariant features among all empirical and imagined examples of suffering and eliminates variations of experience that render it other than suffering, may clarify the invariant core or structure of the experience of suffering. Using imaginative or eidetic variation, researchers systematically vary or change the types of an example under investigation to determine its essential feature, without which the essence would collapse

(Drummond, 2008a). For example, earlier I identified the encounter with the qualities of unboundedness and indeterminacy as essential to suffering. If I imagine an experience of possible suffering that is bounded in some way, such as I know that it will end soon, is the experience still suffering? In other words, when I remove the quality of unboundedness from suffering does its structure collapse so that it is no longer suffering? Eidetic meanings are distinct, however, from empirical exemplifications of the meanings.

Intentional and Essential Structures of Suffering

Starting with Husserl's concepts of intentionality, the individual's life-world and intersubjectivity are central to any understanding of older adults' lived-through suffering. The main research study revealed that the intentional structure of suffering has temporal and developmental moments. In the chapters that follow, I dwell on a temporal moment of the intentional spectrum in which elders participate in the pre-reflective, pre-theoretical, common sense world. While we reflect on and theorize about this world using phenomenological methods, I want to emphasize that older adults themselves inhabit this unthematized world in living their everyday lives, automatically and passively synthesizing knowledge about their social realities and their embedded social cultures.

Husserl's explication of eidetic intuition, when applied to suffering experiences among older adults, allows discernment of the essential structures of suffering among older adults such as loss of agency and loss of the home. Even going beyond the empirical into Husserl's "feigned world" of "eternal truths" (Wertz, 2010), as seen in the great paintings of Picasso, essences can be grasped through artistic presentation that, according to Husserl, has "suggestive power" (Wertz, 2010) or "surplus content" (Barber, 2011) beyond what empirical observation alone can offer us.

Settings

The main, phenomenological study referenced throughout this book was conducted at a care facility in an urban setting. This main study was followed by a second, expanded study that built on the aims of the main study. The follow-up study was conducted at separate and unrelated sites in different geographic communities—one urban and one non-urban—within a region of one state. All three facilities were licensed to provide chronic care. The names and geographic locations of the three facilities are not disclosed to protect the anonymity and privacy of the study participants.

Participant Selection

A purposive sampling selection strategy was used in both studies to select the study participants. "Purposive sampling selection" is the general term used to indicate that the researcher has identified an intentional plan with clear selection criteria to identify cases prior to data collection (Maxwell, 2005). Purposive sampling selection was employed in the main study to select six elderly women participants for in-depth individual interviews. Two men, one elderly and one young-old, were later added to the study sample as comparison cases after approval of an IRB Amendment to the study. Twenty three elderly women and men participants were selected in the follow-up study, for in-depth individual interviews and a more structured interview called a critical incident report, also using purposive sampling selection. (Only the in-depth interviews are drawn upon for the purposes of the narratives in this book.) Purposive sampling selection in both studies aimed for information richness, not population representativeness, and to capture essential patterns across variation (Padgett, 2008; Patton, 2002).

A matrix of demographic characteristics including age, race, ethnicity, religion, income status, and health status was used in both studies to select the participants. Maximal variation in sampling was also sought in the nature and type of significant or major health care decisions that participants had made (in the second study, this field was limited to decisions about pain) (Nelson-Becker, 2006; Padgett, 2008; Patton, 2002).

Eight persons participated in the main study:[2]

- "Angelique" is an 88-year-old black female, widow and mother, who immigrated to America from her native islands. Angelique was first admitted to the short-term rehabilitation unit of the care facility, and several years later transferred to the long-term care unit due to her multiple chronic illness diagnoses including Parkinson's and hypertension, and her functional limitations. She is wheelchair-bound.
- "Camila" is an 87-year-old Latina female, widow with no children, who immigrated to America, and has resided in the long-term care unit of the care facility for over five years. She has diagnoses of hypertension, chronic kidney disease, angina, peripheral vascular disease, and other co-morbid conditions but is ambulatory.
- "Josephina" is a 94-year-old non-Hispanic, white female, widow and mother, who immigrated to America, and has resided in the long-term care unit of the care facility for several years. She has a hypertensive heart, chronic kidney disease, congestive heart failure, diabetes, atrial fibrillation, edema, anemia, dyspnea, and moderate depression. She is wheelchair-bound and requires assistance with ambulation and activities of daily living, but has been evaluated as having no pain.
- "Ruth" is a 90-year-old non-Hispanic, white female, widow and mother, residing in the long-term care unit, and confined to bed.
- "Tawanda" is an 89-year-old black female, widow with no children, residing in the long-term care unit, for several years. She has hypertension and cellulilits, and is wheelchair-bound.
- "Ann" is a 79-year-old non-Hispanic, white female, widow and mother, residing in the long-term care unit, for several years.. She is diabetic, wheelchair-bound, and a very heavy smoker.

- "Alejandro" is a 92-year-old black male, residing in the long-term care unit, with chronic obstructive pulmonary disease and renal failure.
- "Harvey" is a 55-year-old single, non-Hispanic, white male, diabetic, with a partial leg amputation, admitted to the long-term care unit of the care facility. Harvey is confined to bed most of the time.

The expanded aims of the second, follow-up study were to: i) describe lived experiences of pain from the perspectives of older adults and their family members in their life-historical contexts, and deepen understanding of their meanings and ethical implications for decision making; ii) identify the distinct structures of pain and suffering experiences, and the relationship of pain to suffering experience; and iii) explore what seriously ill older adults want at the end of life as they live through pain and make decisions about their health and health care, especially in light of frequent incongruence between clinical data including goals of care and assessments, and persons' life-historical experience. In addition, the second study focused on the non-linear, dialectical relationship between older adults' decision making and pain experiences and outcomes, including the role and effectiveness of processes of decision making in changing or modifying older adults' pain, and the relationship of such processes to self-efficacy, agency, decisional conflict, and pain outcomes. As the second study developed, these aims were expanded to include investigation of elders' chronic pain experiences in a sub-sample of older adults with diabetes and chronic wounds.

The following seven individuals among twenty-three participants from the follow-up study[3] are referenced in the chapter narratives:

- "Peter" is a 62-year-old black male, diabetic, admitted to the care facility, post-surgery with complex wounds, dehydration, and weight loss, and discharged to a lower level of care after three months.
- "Michael" is a 72-year-old non-Hispanic, white male, diabetic, admitted to the care facility with complex wounds, and discharged to a lower level of care after several months..
- "Barney" is a 75-year-old non-Hispanic, white male, diabetic, admitted to the care facility with complex wounds and renal failure.
- "Peggy" is an 84-year-old black female, admitted to the care facility with a diagnosis of Parkinson's disease, and is a heavy smoker. Peggy uses a wheelchair for mobility in the care facility.
- "Bernadette" is a 96-year-old non-Hispanic, white female, diabetic, admitted to the care facility, post-hospitalization and as a transfer from another facility. She has congestive heart failure, shortness of breath, but reports no pain. Bernadette has aided ambulation.
- "Virginia" is a 75-year-old non-Hispanic, white female, admitted to the care facility with diagnoses of Parkinson's disease, hypertension, and chronic leg pain. Virginia ambulates with the aid of a walker.
- "Chris" is a young-old, non-Hispanic, white male, admitted to the care facility with metastatic cancer, confined to bed most of the time.

Both studies were submitted to and approved by the Fordham University Institutional Review Board (IRB). All participants in the studies signed informed consents also approved by the Fordham University IRB.

The anonymity of the participants in the chapter narratives is protected through the use of alias names, and intentional non-disclosure of specific information that might lead to unintended identification such as place of origin, dates of admission, and names and geographic locations of facility sites.

Data Collection

I as the researcher (and principal investigator in the second study), conducted and completed all phases of data collection and data analysis in both studies that are made a part of the chapter narratives in this book. The primary form of data collection in both the main and follow-up study was open-ended, in-depth interviews. My ethnographic observations as researcher were also a form of data collection for the purposes of these narratives. In the main study, I spent six months at the research site, and in the follow-up study, was at each of the respective research sites for approximately six months. This kind of "embeddedness" and prolonged engagement at the sites, in a non-staff capacity, strengthen the trustworthiness of the data.

Limitations

A limitation of the main and follow-up studies is the relatively small sample size, although the studies aimed for information richness and not population representativeness. Findings are not generalizable in the way that findings from a quantitative study with probability sampling would be. However, there are some contexts in which the findings may be generalized, which I will address more fully in the last chapter. For example, the findings overall may be generalized to seriously ill elders in care facilities. The invariant dimensions of suffering experience, which were found to have high-level generality, may be applicable to all seriously ill persons.

There are certain limitations related to the study participants. The participants' illness and suffering burdens may have compromised their willingness to give the researcher full access to their lived experiences, especially if there were a problem of collapsed agency. The participants may also have experienced limited concerns about facility or health care professional access to their confidential information, even though I as the researcher completed the full informed consent process with each one of them prior to commencement of the interviews, and regularly reminded them of their confidentiality and privacy protections. Participants' language in certain cases may also constitute a limitation on the findings. The aboriginal language and expressions of the participants have been preserved and are integrated into the narratives. In certain individual cases and in a small number of instances, participants' language expressions and meanings were difficult to understand without looking at context.

Maternal Affordances in Human Development from Birth to Death: Ground for Ethical Provision of Care in Serious Illness and at End of Life

From Freud to Winnicott, and among the many developmental and theoretical psychologists and theoreticians in other disciplines who have followed and advanced their work, the study of Maternal experience and Maternal care has been a central focus in understanding infant and early childhood development, including capacity for moral intuition and emotion (Bloom, 2013). Winnicott's (1965) construct of the Maternal "holding environment" has also been used in multiple contexts of human development, experience, and relational care, such as psychoanalysis (Neuman, 2013; Orange, 2011; Slochower, 2014; Starr, 2008; Stern, 1985; Summers, 2013; Wertz, 1981), and in feminist care ethics (Roberts & Reich, 2002; Rogers, 2009) to describe the constituents of the Maternal attitude and Maternal dimensions of existence essential to care provision. In the mental health services arena, Larry Davidson (2003) has shed light on the role of institutions in patterns of recidivism among persons with serious mental illness who turn to institutions seeking the food, comfort, security and social support not available to them in the community. Other researchers studying schizophrenia have identified certain similar patterns (Kamens, Forgione, Minahan, & Driggs, 2014). While this evidence runs counter to Goffman's "total institutions" (Goffman, 1961) and Foucault's "panopticism" (Foucault, 1995) theories, it also suggests that there may be more than one type of environmental care provision, or that environments are experienced differently by different persons. Even in light of this established body of work on care ethics and care environments, little has been written or adduced in the way of evidence about the role of the Maternal and the Maternal process of "holding" and care provision in the context of palliative and end-of-life care, and impact upon the health and well-being of seriously ill persons, especially since the early work of Cicely Saunders (Saunders, 2011) and Colin Murray Parkes in developing support programs for the dying and bereaved in hospice (Bretherton, 1992). The main and follow-up studies discussed in this book identify the essential constituents of the Maternal and Maternal Affordances in suffering experience in the contexts of chronic, serious and life-limiting illness, and the empathic Maternal care being sought by seriously ill elders. They illustrate the relationship of these constituents to each other, to Maternal experience as a whole over the lifespan, especially in the midst of suffering, and to development from birth to death within the nested interpersonal, family, and larger systems of community in which the suffering elder is situated.

In phenomenological psychology, one of the most significant contributions to an understanding of suffering among older adults goes back to Freud (1948, 1952, 1954, 1965) and the psychoanalysts and developmental psychologists who followed him—Ainsworth and Bowlby (Ainsworth & Bowlby, 1965; Bowlby, 1957, 1958, 1960, 1965, 1989), Winnicott (1965), Guntrip (1985), and DeRobertis (2010). Freud understood something primal in the origins and meanings of suffering that remains just as essential to the flourishing of older adults as to infants: the primal Maternal relationship—also recognized by Alfred Schütz (1966). This primal Maternal relationship revealed itself in this study of elderly persons in care facilities as an essential structure in the life-historical narratives of elder suffering. Why would it make sense that the Maternal would be thematized in these narratives, even for elderly women who themselves had never been mothers, or for older men?

The Maternal Ground, as I have named it, encompassed Maternal dimensions of existence that formed the most vital aspects of human development in the lived past of these frail elders living in facility environments: holding, feeding and nurture, relational intimacy, loving care, the provision of a welcoming home, comfort and security, and the capacity for generative, self-actualizing agency. These experiences that are reactivated and show themselves in later life have been passively synthesized and built up over the elders' life course at the pre-reflective level, and retained by elders as part of their common sense lives and understandings, resurfacing after their traumatic transition to the facility. The transfer to an institutional setting marks a disruption in elders' life-world existence and "continuity of being" (Winnicott, 1965, p. 54; Wertz, 1981), but it also creates a possibility for transformative development. In certain cases in the main study, the common sense shared understanding of the Maternal took on linguistic and cultural meanings that were specific to a cultural subgroup. However, the general structure of suffering that proved invariant was the loss of Maternal Foundations and the loss of participation in the passively synthesized common sense life these foundations supported—comparable to some extent to the aspects of dysfunction called "ipseity disorder" found in schizophrenia as described by Louis Sass and colleagues (Sass, Parnas, & Zahavi, 2011).

The parallels between suffering experience and disorders of the self among those with a diagnosis of schizophrenia inform our understanding of suffering. The central feature of "ipseity" disorder, as described by Sass, Parnas, and Zahavi (2011, p. 1), that appears in suffering experience is disintegration, or the threat of such disintegration of the unified, "core" self, such that experience of the self as one in the same self in a temporal moment becomes fractured (ibid., 2011, p. 7). There are two prominent manifestations of this disorder of the self that appear in elders' suffering experience. The first is what the researchers call "diminished self-affection" or failed or distorted awareness of the unified self; the second is "hyperreflexivity" or heightened forms of self-consciousness that disrupt the pre-reflective, common sense life (ibid., 2011, p. 7). In practical terms, these aspects of suffering are translated into profound losses of Maternal Foundations and agency for the seriously ill elderly person who is hospitalized or residing in a care facility. It is here, in the complex nexus or "enclave" (Schütz, 1973) of suffering as it intersects with the Maternal and disorders of the self that we discern the Maternal as an *eidos* of significance in and of itself that has implications for human development, self-actualization, and mature self-identity. This understanding of disintegration and to some extent, loss of self and self-identity at the *pre-reflective* level, are findings that run counter to conventional understandings about experiences of suffering described in the literature that view suffering as only a passive undergoing. I include these parallels to self-experience disorders for the purposes of description and eidetic analysis of essential features of suffering. I make no commentary or draw no conclusions about the clinical significance of these findings either for suffering elders or individuals with diagnoses of schizophrenia, except to suggest tentatively that one possible interpretation of these data is that schizophrenia is a form of suffering and therefore shares in common with suffering these essential features. However, not all suffering experiences would be experiences of schizophrenia as other essential dimensions of schizophrenia are absent. Suffering too has other qualities or essential constituents that go beyond the self. These constituents are located at the nexus of the self, the intentional structure of consciousness, and the intentional world. Here I am proposing that the experience of suffering is delimited not only by the self as existing in the world, but by the capacity of the self and a mature consciousness to transcend themselves.

The syncretic state of early childhood development, in which children form their beliefs and basic understanding of the world, may re-appear at other stages in life (Merleau-Ponty, 1964). Suffering elders may be described as embedded in a type of syncretism in their caregiving relationships and care environments, through which they seek the caring hospitality and welcome of the Maternal home. Even their postural stance toward the world, as reflected in their intentional bodily relation—what Merleau-Ponty calls "operative intentionality"—may indicate their high state of suffering, dependency, or longing for Maternal embrace. It is at this pre-reflective, operative intentionality level that the disorders of the self occur (Sass, Parnas, & Zahavi, 2011). For example, it is very common to see older adults confined to wheelchairs, especially in care facilities, and this confinement in many ways defines these elders' bodily relation to the world, a world shrunken both spatially and temporally, in which they are frequently cut off from any meaningful social engagement. More specifically, the phenomenology of perception elaborated by Merleau-Ponty (1962) and others helps to illuminate questions of epistemology or knowledge of the other as they relate to suffering, and strengthen the case for the Maternal as a ground of subject-world intentional connection. Non-linguistic symbols, such as the work of Picasso or the intersubjective encounter in musical experience as described by Schutz, also permit unmediated openness to reality (Husserl, 1913/1982; Wertz, 2010), in this case the reality of suffering. In other words, it is not necessary for a suffering elder to say, "See me, I am suffering," in order to be perceived by others, intuitively and automatically, as a being-in-suffering.

Merleau-Ponty's achievements in undermining the significance of mind–body dualisms rooted in Cartesianism that result in polarizing the mind and body are relevant to studies of suffering because they bring to prominence the role of the lived body in human experience and the body's inseparability from psychic and spiritual life. They also highlight the inadequacy of approaches to illness that reduce human beings to mere homunculi (Morrissey, 2014b). His notion of the directedness of the body toward the world illuminates the pre-reflective movement of the body in grasping objects in the world and in locating its postural stance in relation to the world. This is a directedness that is not-language dependent, but occurs at the pre-verbal level in the lived body's field of existence. In *The Child's Relations with Others*, Merleau-Ponty (1964) describes the state of syncretic sociability in which early Maternal–child relations characterized primarily by the non-differentiated identity of the child with her/his mother lie at the basis of human development from its earliest stages and throughout the life course. The mother's holding and cradling of the infant, acts of nurture through breastfeeding, and the infant's latching on to the mother's breast (Ryan, Todres, & Alexander, 2010), are examples of syncretic sociability at the level of primal and pre-reflective psychological development. According to Merleau-Ponty, this type of syncretic state and unmediated experience can occur at other times in human experience, such as in illness through a process of non-differentiated alliance with a caregiver or embedded in a caregiving environment, and in this way found intersubjective understanding.[4]

Elders' interests in, and retentions of the Maternal dimensions of existence, are thus not regressive by virtue of the essential nature of the Maternal alone. The Maternal experience is generative while also protective. In suffering elders, there is a drive or projective, life-force movement toward futural horizons in the later life course. For example, suffering among seriously ill older adults at the end of life motivated older adults' desire to seek empathic, Maternal care in their relationships with caregivers. Gonzalez Sanders & Fortinsky (2012) have described the elder–caregiver relationship, in particular in cases of elder dementia, as a symbiosis. While the elders who are the subjects of these narratives all met eligibility criteria for decision-making capacity, the research findings suggest that if there were such an elder–caregiver symbiosis, it would be a generative symbiosis and not a destructive one. Although there may be a re-enactment of retained or assimilated experiences of dependency or attachment in elders' life-affirming, care-seeking drive for well-being, this movement is neither a regression nor a return to this earlier state, but ultimately the generative act of an autonomous person whose intentionalities and interests motivate development (Morrissey, 2011b). The care-seeking movement that manifests itself in elders' generative acts may not always be linear. Rather, it may manifest itself in cycles of latency and growth. The meanings that such generative movement and acts have for elders may vary in each individual elder's own experience. Maternal Affordances in elder suffering and care-seeking, as in infant and early childhood development, are therefore not reducible to regression or satisfaction of basic needs. They are opportunities for fruitful action. In multiple ways, Maternal Affordances in suffering experiences, through passive syntheses, make available the possibility for transformative development experiences of agency and spiritual flourishing.

Seismic shifts in social relationships, social roles, and social contexts play an essential part in the suffering experienced by elders. Alfred Schütz (1951, 1962, 1964, 1966, 1967, 1973, 1996), who greatly expanded our understanding of social reality, locates the origin of intersubjectivity in the primal Maternal relationship. In the concept of the "*We-relation*," Schütz advanced the notion of intersubjective experience. Richard Zaner (2002), in a rich analysis of intersubjectivity, reflects on the meaning of the "We-relation" and the significance of Schutz's writing on "being born and brought up by mothers" for understanding his conceptualization of intersubjectivity (p. 16). Zaner tentatively proposes that Schutz conceptualizes intersubjectivity and empathy as given in the primal Maternal relation:

> We may then be able to suggest, albeit in the most tentative manner here, that being human is indeed truly a gift: being human is being gifted both with my life and the sense of myself as having to be achieved. The primal Other, mother, 'gifts' me with myself (gift of life from pregnancy, birth); and later, gifts me with herself (through words; stories). Being born is accordingly constitutive of what and who I, any I, am; I am not merely, then, a "being-toward-death," but even more fundamentally a "being-from-birth"... I am indebted for my being to the Other (mother first of all), and responsible then for proper recognition of that and of becoming myself... done within the nexus of growing old together.
>
> (Zaner, 2002, p. 17)

The implications of this analysis of Schützian intersubjectivity for seriously ill elderly persons struggling with the experiences and consequences of aging and chronic illnesses, as well as end-of-life choices and decisions, are crucial. Schütz described the primordial experiences of relational encounter and intimacy in the Maternal relation and birth: "As long as man is born of woman, intersubjectivity and the we-relationship will be the foundation for all other categories of human existence" (Schütz 1957/1966, p. 82). And he stated further, "As long as human beings are not concocted like homunculi in retorts but are born and brought up by mothers, the sphere of the 'We' will be naively presupposed" (Schütz 1962 [1942], p. 168).

Schütz (1962) also advanced a notion of multiple realities that can be located in "enclaves" or "finite provinces" of meaning—subsets of the much vaster social reality—enclosed within one another. These diverse provinces of meaning intersect yet retain their phenomenological identity, some more intensely than others. Examples of Schüztian enclaves have been described and found in the world of working, dreaming, literature, religion (Schutz, 1973; Barber, 2014), and in the essential constituents of Maternal care experienced in the intensely lived experiences of illness and suffering (Morrissey, 2011), as well as more generally, in caring relationships (Rogers, 2009). Here I advance a more comprehensive notion of the Maternal as itself a finite province of meaning, and a "paramount reality," as Schutz used this term to describe the "archetype" of reality (although Schutz himself identified the world of working as the archetype) (Barber, 2014). While Schütz never quite came to terms with Husserl on how intersubjectivity works (Barber, 2011; Zaner, 2002), intersubjectivity is central to the problem of knowledge in elder care. Unlike Husserl, Schütz believed that intersubjectivity is a given, not a problem (Zaner, 2002). Based on analyses of Schütz's writing by both Zaner (2002) and Barber (2011), it is clear that Schütz located intersubjectivity in the common sense world, and the origin of intersubjectivity in the primal Maternal relation. In "Making Music Together," one of Schütz's most famous essays, he drew on music and its polythetic design to show how reality is encountered and directly accessed in the "mutual tuning-in relationship" (Schutz, 1951, p. 79). Barber (2010) helps to illuminate the nature of Schütz's "mutual tuning-in relationship" by spelling out that this relationship has priority over, comes before, and founds communication and expression. Barber (2014) elaborates further on certain aspects of the non-working finite province of meaning, as disclosed in literature and religion, that "resist pragmatism… by: 1) the way it organizes the world about another point of orientation; 2) its awareness of the limited ability of the ego's power to bring transcendences within reach insofar as another power underpins the ego's exercise of its own power; 3) its placing the fundamental anxiety and the relevances it shapes in a non-pragmatic context; 4) its refocusing on frequently overlooked unique and atypical aspects of experience; and 5) its attention to aspects of intersubjective relationships, which the world of working does not allow us the leisure to consider" (p. 18). It is proposed, however tentatively, that the Maternal, like religion, is a non-working finite province of meaning not dominated by pragmatism and characterized by the foregoing features. This understanding of the Maternal has important implications for the study of older adults and their suffering experience because of the possibility the Maternal finite province of meaning affords to transcend suffering.

Suffering as Ethical Encounter

Intersubjective understanding makes possible an ethical encounter in which the subject recognizes the other as someone like "me" who experiences pain and suffers like "me". In this encounter, I gain immediate access to the person's experiences through the mechanisms of empathy, self-transposition, and passive syntheses. I know the other as a suffering other like myself without having to make any deductive inferences and without having to engage in any reflection. This encounter occurs below the level of theory or inference.

Genetic phenomenological analysis helps to illuminate these origins of suffering. The primordial origins of suffering in human development go all the way down to the Maternal relation—both in Maternal-fetal development, ruptured by the discontinuity of being born into a world of others (Wertz, 1981), and later in the Maternal–child relations described by Merleau-Ponty as a state of undifferentiated syncretic sociability as discussed above. In studying experiences such as health, illness, moral agency, and decision making, phenomenology seeks to comprehend the world in terms of its origins, its concealed horizons, its possibility, and even the transcendence of possibility. Maternal dimensions of existence, in building knowledge of the experience of suffering—a central problem in health care and bioethics, help to inform understanding of creative fidelity to the *other*.

The salience of the encounter with the suffering elder as an ethical encounter is critical. Levinas (1969) correctly places the ethical relation in the pre-theoretical, pre-reflective, and pre-ontological realm. The call of the suffering elder *other* is unquestionably a summons to ethical responsibility. Likewise, the work of John

Drummond (2008), and contemporary political scientists such as Matthew O'Brien (2011), show clearly that moral experience and moral decision making are embedded in the common sense life, in social practices. This brings us back full circle to a focus on the pre-reflective, temporal life-world in which elders in their everyday experience.

Social and Developmental Aspects of Suffering: From Losses of Maternal Foundations to Strivings for Well-Being

In the main research study of suffering among frail elderly care facility residents, the major findings entailed the identification of social and developmental aspects of suffering and the loss of Maternal Foundations in the transition to the care facility. The first temporal moment in development, which I call the Maternal Ground, endowed elderly persons with the means to forge vital connections with the lived world and to engage creatively with the elder's own radical freedom. The key pillars of the Maternal Ground are empathy, receptivity, care, and the generative possibility for development.

Interpreters of Husserl and Schütz, who differ in their views of how empathy works, have developed multiple approaches to empathy. Michael Barber (2010) provides a clear account of empathy, drawing parallels between Husserl and Schütz and giving prominence to the role of genetic phenomenology in the structure of empathy, once again locating this essentially human experience in the pre-reflective, common sense life, and in passive syntheses below the level of theory or inferential thought. Barber (2010) explains the idea of the bodily transference in passive synthesis of the "animate organism" to the other as described by Husserl:

> Here I will articulate what I take to be three reasons why Husserl in his Nachlass writings has such confidence in the analogical apperceptive transfer of the sense "lived body" to the other and why he believes that the transfer cannot be blocked due to the lack of original experience of the other. The first has to do with overwhelming number and pervasiveness of ways in which similarity grounds the transference—something that becomes clearer in the three volumes on intersubjectivity than in the highly condensed argument of the Cartesian Meditations. There is first of all a similarity between the physical appearances of my body and the other to whom the sense "lived body" is transferred, especially our various organs, but this similarity is not only a matter of physical resemblance, as if we were merely things similar to each other, but it also has to do with how those organs function as part of a whole bodily organ system that functions like our bodily system, as Husserl suggest in his discussion of how we observe the other governing (Walten) in his or her body in the Cartesian Meditations. Higher species, such as apes, remind me of myself and evoke the transference of "lived body" insofar as they possess and function with hands and feet, organs for grasping things (Greiforganen), as even lower species can do insofar as they exhibit sensitivity

in their skin and appropriate reaction-movements, such as the quivering of the skin when pricked, as happens with us, or the wrinkling of the forehead upon being touched or struck.[vii] The behavior of the other lived body can elicit the transfer insofar as I am reminded of my lived body by: its valuing; striving; acting; grasping according to right or left, before or after; shoving; bumping up against; touching; carrying; doing; suffering; being pained by bright sunlight; acting; reacting; retreating before an object of fear; being attracted to food; eating; producing the violent movements and shrieking voice that are indicative of anger; achieving ends; seeing; and judging or speaking out (the latter two being particularly human).

(Barber, 2010[5])

Barber (2013) expounds further on passive transfers between animate organisms:

Another factor that Schütz seems to overlook is the extensive similarities present between animate organisms. Beyond the similarity existing between my hand and another human being's hand, various species possess other features that passively evoke the transfer, such as the hands or feet of primates, similar to my own; organs used for grasping things, as crabs' claws; and the sensitivity of skin and correlative reaction-movements, as when a worm withdraws from being pricked or an animal's forehead wrinkles when it is pained. The assorted behaviors of another lived body can elicit the transfer insofar as I am reminded of my lived body by the other's: valuing; striving; acting; grasping according to right or left, before or after; shoving; bumping up against; touching; carrying; doing; suffering; being pained by bright sunlight; acting; reacting; retreating before an object of fear; being attracted to food; eating; producing the agitated movements and shrieking voice indicative of anger; achieving ends; seeing; and judging or speaking out (the latter two being particularly human).

However, it is not merely the having of organs similar to mine or the sharing of many similar features, though, that evokes the transfer of "animate organism" to the other. Once can imagine a decapitated head with its eyes frozen open, and one might not make the transfer—in fact such an experience can be extremely uncomfortable insofar as one notices eyes, ears, and a mouth like one's own, but no motion at all. The head does not exhibit animation, and this strangeness or even eeriness upsets the usually immediate transfer of the sense "animate organism" to which I would be inclined on the basis of physical features similar to my own. What is further necessary is that body resembling mine in its eyes, ears, mouth, or mien also appear as single, unified, whole organism in which another subject governs or holds sway (*walten*). As examples of animals holding sway in their animate organism, one might think of the dog playing with the newspaper in coordination with my extending the paper toward it or the fish softly waving its fins and tail in such a way as to maintain a stable position in the water so that it might be able to look at me.

(pp. 320–321)

Many aspects of the lived body that Barber enumerates and describes in the foregoing passages are present and in play in the narratives of suffering elders presented in the chapters that follow, and remind the "second person" of his or her own lived body. It is argued that this transference of the sense lived body through analogy lays the ground for empathic access to elders' suffering experience. This view has also been challenged, however. Zahavi (2001) has suggested that empathy may not be central to intersubjectivity. Rather, he has advanced a synthesis of competing theories and identified the pre-linguistic character of intersubjectivity, and the triangulation of self, others and world as distinctive features of the phenomenolgoical approach to intersubjectivity. These very same features are also essential constituents of the Maternal.

One of the most exciting research findings was that, in the midst of immense suffering and illness burden, frail elders still struggled to achieve well-being. How did this intentionality arise? The analysis showed that these intentionalities were founded upon re-enactments of the Maternal dimensions of existence, and moved beyond re-enactments into generative, self-actualizing mechanisms of self-efficacy and agency. These very sick, frail elders displayed agency in the common sense habitual tasks of living—such as making their beds, going to meals, and praying the rosary—as well as making themselves heard as full participants in their own care planning whenever they felt marginalized. Their agency was most evident, however, in the areas of faith, spiritual growth and flourishing, reflecting a transcendent movement toward hope and the future. Marcel (1962) wrote that hope "resides in the creative voluntary act" and the faculty of reason [is] distinct" (p. 65). It is found in the presence of faith, fidelity, and what he calls "disposability." (Marcel, 1949, p. 69).

In the face of the "ultimate boundary of death," as Schütz calls it, or the "fundamental anxiety" of death (Schütz, 1964, p. 82; Zaner, 2002, p. 14), there is the possibility that receptivity and availability, a letting go of omnipotence and control, and an acceptance of frailty, vulnerability, and dependency in a community with others may be the ultimate expressions of freedom, faith, and hope in growing old. Echoing Levinas, preventing elders from growing old and dying alone in states of social isolation, impoverishment, desolation and despair is a shared ethical responsibility.

My research on suffering among frail elders builds upon a legacy of scholarship from Freud and Winnicott to Wertz and Barber. Drawing on the research findings presented in the chapter narratives of the book, I suggest that the Maternal Ground and its essential constituents are central to understanding elders' life-historical experiences of suffering and care-seeking intentionalities, desires, and behaviors, to fostering elders' full agentic freedom and fidelity to their socially constituted life-worlds, meanings and relationships with others and, most importantly, to their flourishing and the possibility of hope even in the last days of their lives. The narrative accounts of elders in the midst of suffering through serious illness illuminate and give life to their multiple meanings of freedom, fidelity, and faith.

Conclusion

The structure of Maternal Affordances, and Maternal care as "environmental provision" (Winnicott, 1965) for those who are seriously ill and suffering will be elaborated in the chapters that follow. Maternal generosity and relational intimacy, unconditional loving care and touch, empathy, fidelity, a receptive and protective welcoming home that is palliative and assures well-being, and desire and generative possibility for development are essential constituents of the Maternal that must be translated into meaningful care provision in a holding environment designed to fit the care-seeking needs of seriously ill older adults and at the same time create a space for their growth and development, in particular, a movement toward fulfilling agency and spiritual transformation. The process of development in infancy from total dependency to transitional object relations, and finally disentanglement from Maternal care can be traced to and paralleled in the generative psychological, emotional, and social process that occurs in the progression from serious illness to end of life. The central role of Maternal Affordances and care at the end of life mirrors the Maternal environment in relation to the infant: the integrating function of the holding environment is a ground not only of total support and palliation for the dying person who is living through pain and suffering and calling for the other, but also a ground of final and inexorable processes of life integration, personal and interpersonal reconciliation, and ultimately, final separation and disentanglement from all intentional, social relations with the world and others in the world that signal the impingement of death.

Finally, the implications of these findings for improving care practices and designing palliative environments, and their impact upon public health ethics and bioethical inquiry will be discussed. The essentially ethical nature of the Maternal relation and Maternal care obligation to the other will also be probed, as they concern appropriate ethics education for all health and human service professionals involved in care provision.

Notes

1   Bioethics, 4E. © 2014 Gale, a part of Cengage Learning, Inc., p. 292. Reproduced by permission. www.cengage.com/permissions
2   Morrissey, M. B. (2011a). "Suffering and Decision Making Among Seriously Ill Elderly Women." Unpublished Dissertation, Fordham University.
3   Morrissey, M. B., Wertz, F. J., Comfort, C., Jennings, B., Mendell, J., & Leach, T. (2014). Pain and Decision Making Among Seriously Ill Older Adults. Unpublished study. Funded by the Translational Institute for Pain in Later Life.
4   Bioethics, 4E. © 2014 Gale, a part of Cengage Learning, Inc., pp. 2392–2393. Reproduced by permission. www.cengage.com/permissions
5   Page number in published work not available.

2 The Narrative of Angelique
Maternal Affordances and Maternal Grace

In this chapter, I introduce the story of Angelique, a frail, seriously ill 88-year-old woman living in a care facility. I first started seeing Angelique in the spring of 2010. Angelique's family had placed her in a care facility after deciding that she was no longer able to live independently in her own home. Angelique had multiple chronic illnesses—Parkinson's disease, hypertension, and mild depression—and was wheelchair-bound most of the time. I developed a very good rapport with Angelique over the six months that I visited her to conduct interviews for my study. She was always happy to see me, and each successive time I came to visit her she felt more comfortable with me. It was not until the early fall, though, near the end of our visits, that she shared with me the most meaningful aspects of her life history, particularly her early life growing up in her native islands, her coming to America, and her important life events—marriage, children, working, and her relationships with family.

Angelique's narrative as presented in this chapter is a genetic phenomenological analysis of her experiences and how they were constituted, going back to their beginnings, and a synthesis of the constituents of Angelique's individual structure of suffering, based upon her own descriptions. In this narrative, the Maternal dimensions of existence emerge as the ground of Angelique's most meaningful experiences in her later life as a resident of a chronic care facility.

First Temporal Moment: Maternal Ground and Genetic Constitution of Empathy

Angelique's individual structure of suffering is formed upon a ground of essential aspects of the Maternal: empathy, receptivity, generosity and relational intimacy, unconditional loving care and touch, fidelity, a receptive and protective welcoming home that is palliative and assures well-being, desire, and generative possibility for development. The primordial interpersonal relationship Angelique experienced in Maternal dimensions of existence drives her call for nurturance and her empathic, care-seeking behavior when she is no longer able to care for herself. The Maternal Relation lays the foundation for the development of a desire for sociality, meaning and fulfillment, and empathic care. In interviews with Angelique, Angelique describes dimensions of a Maternal Ground and the meanings it has for her in her experiences of suffering. Through end-of-life illness and decision making in the care facility setting, Angelique experiences the Maternal Ground as a well-spring of intersubjectivity, interconnectedness, and interembodied care.

Empathy is a core, essential, and invariant constituent of the Maternal for Angelique, with its roots in her early childhood development. Angelique experiences empathy through intuitive "seeing" of the Maternal in her recollections of past "essentially actual experiences" such as her internal perceptions of her own feelings (Barber, 2012; Schutz, 1962, p. 53) associated with Maternal care and interembodiment, or through immediate and automatic passive syntheses of experiences that are brought to bear now at the pre-reflective level, but occurred as passive syntheses in her infancy or early childhood and have been built up over time (Barber, 2012). Interembodiment in the syncretic Maternal state is characterized by non-differentiation—in its own various stages. This non-differentiation does not suggest that the infant is not over time developing an individuated consciousness pre-reflectively, but rather is doing so in a "holding" environment (Winnicott, 1965) that is supportive, protective and performing integrating functions that the infant cannot yet perform on her/his own. This non-differentiation is not one of identity, but principally involves the unmediated experience of embodied care in a totally supportive environment. This is consistent with Michael Barber's (2012) description of passive syntheses in infancy, which according to Barber go beyond Merleau-Ponty's understanding at the time he was writing of how these processes work. Merleau-Ponty correctly identified the syncretic state that may appear at other times in the life course, but did not correctly describe the content of the state in that he did not fully appreciate that differentiation of identity does occur in the syncretic state. It is dependence on the care environment and the experience of unmediated care that I abstract from Merleau-Ponty's descriptions that are most relevant to understanding of suffering and recollection and re-enactment of Maternal dimensions of existence in elders' later life course.

For Angelique, these descriptions of interembodiment and Maternal body extend beyond the physical to shared understandings and shared meanings, which are assimilated in Angelique's consciousness. Her past experiences of being in relation, interembodied care, and Maternal roles, such as the "housedness" provided in the Maternal dwelling and the nourishment provided in Maternal feeding, in part constitute these shared meanings and understandings. Angelique brings to bear in the present temporal moment her recollections and passive syntheses of Maternal experience that become a ground of her intentionalities, desires, and agency in her current situation in the care facility. These assimilations become part of a temporal horizon of experience and embedded agency that help Angelique to cope with the suffering she experiences in the care facility through her end-of-life decision making.

Elderly individuals may experience empathy in a variety of different ways, however, within pervasive meanings of the Maternal. For example, dimensions of empathic understanding, which are essential to the Maternal, may reveal themselves in experiences of art, music, or the mystical. The mystical and Maternal character of Angelique's faith in God provides her with spiritual nurturance and support, as well as comfort and security. Angelique also experiences interembodiment and Maternal care through a sense of community, both from the community in which she was embedded in her native islands and the community she hopes for in her future life. The essential constituents of the Maternal relate to each other dynamically and form a unified Maternal Ground of experience in end-of-life illness.

Maternal Attitude and Affordances

Maternal generosity, relational intimacy, receptivity and care

From Angelique's earliest recollections and earliest assimilated history, the Maternal dimensions of existence have constituted her life-world. Throughout the narrative, Angelique makes multiple references to the Maternal aspects of experience. She hearkens back to her early life in her native islands, in her home of origin with her mother and siblings, where she was happy to be nourished emotionally and physically, enjoying everyday things like cooking and sleeping. She doesn't remember her father, but she recalls her grandmother and great-grandmother clearly, recounting her shared intimacy with them in Maternal relationships. Angelique recognizes the personal significance of the Maternal care and support she received at that developmental moment:

> Yes, I had a home in the islands. Nothing great about it, my home in the islands. I'm glad we had a place to sleep. We had a place to sleep and were able to cook. And my mother fed us. I lived with [my] mother and the other children, but not my father. My father died pretty young, because I've never seen his face. No, I never saw him. I saw my grandmother, my father's mother, but I've never seen my father's face. But his mother, now, I know. I know my father's mother, and his grandmother. ... I remember quite a bit about them. ... My grandmother took us to school.

The intricacies of Angelique's experiences of suffering and decision making in the care facility begin here in her native islands with a Maternal Ground that is both frame of reference and a horizon (Geniusas, 2010), that fully implicates all possible fruitions that arise from it as the origin of intersubjective experience. Angelique references and brings her past life-course Maternal and developmental experiences to bear in her end-of-life illness and suffering.

Angelique elaborates on Maternal intimacy she experienced in describing the practice of island mothers' breastfeeding their babies for an extended time. Through this experience of nursing, Angelique assimilates the meanings of interembodied Maternal care:

Back in the islands, they all had to nurse the baby. Sometimes up to a year, they're still nursing, yeah. Yes, my mother did that, nursed the babies. Yes, till they were older. That was the custom there. And the next custom is a little thin porridge in a bottle. And I started to give my granddaughter, my Magda, cereal in her cup, figuring that when my daughter Marge finished nursing the baby and they put the baby to sleep, she wouldn't be so hungry.

This ongoing nourishment of babies with breast milk and later with porridge is central to Angelique's experience of a Maternal Ground. For Angelique, the process of nourishing extends beyond bodily feeding to a form of embodied care.

These descriptions of Angelique's early life experiences exemplify the phenomenal experience of syncretic sociability of mother and child, a state of relational intimacy with the mother in which the child, in the very early stages of development, is not reflectively aware of the environment in which she is being held and in that sense, may be viewed as in a non-differentiated state from the Maternal holding environment and Maternal care. In describing the Maternal feeding and care she received as a child, Angelique certainly recollects her lived experience of being nurtured by her mother through the act of feeding, but in the larger context of the ongoing provision of nourishment and care essential to her growth, development, and well-being as an infant, as a young child, and even as an adult. This Maternal feeding and nourishment are not reducible to bodily nourishment or satisfaction of basic needs alone. I shall call a Maternal surplus that exceeds satisfaction of basic needs "Maternal Affordances." Angelique's rich descriptions about knowing her paternal grandmother and great-grandmother enact relational intimacies for her that constitute a core meaning of the Maternal dimensions of her existence. Her loss of these Maternal Foundations and relational intimacy on which her life once rested become a source of pain and suffering for Angelique when she transitions to the care facility. The Maternal Ground becomes thematic and central to her as she attempts to envision what she needs and strives to attain in the reinstatement of Maternal security. I want to be clear here that Angelique never loses the very Maternal Ground itself, but "Maternal Foundations"—the term I use to describe all experiences and meanings that are built on the Maternal Ground or spring from it. The Maternal Ground itself is always given and present, in the world, although may not be visible or seen by the suffering elder. This Maternal state of givenness, "Maternal Grace," echoes Karl Rahner's (1967) notion of grace as that which self-communicates itself in the lived world of ordinary experience. It is a condition of possibility for all autonomous and creative, generative acts of freedom.

The processes of feeding and nourishment, and relational intimacy in the Maternal system, take on a special significance for Angelique in her social and cultural context. The larger meanings implicit in the experiences she describes are manifold. The mother's unconditional generosity in offering milk to the baby, the baby's desire for the mother's milk, the rooting for milk at the mother's nipple, and the mother's loving care of the baby and the child all forge the relational bond between the child Angelique and her mother. The materiality of the mother's milk itself is constitutive of the interembodied care of the Maternal system, and is made manifest and re-enacted in seeking and receiving soothing care, comfort, security, and guidance in response to distress and dislocation. Angelique's first and primordial interpersonal relation forms within this context of Maternal dimensions of feeding, care, nurture—the satisfaction of basic and developmental needs, and attachment. Various forms of this interpersonal union, syncretic sociability or attachment will appear in Angelique's adult relationships and end-of-life illness experiences, through primary passivity or association that occurs within Angelique's own consciousness and secondary passive associations with culture and community (Drummond, 2008b), especially in her frail dependent state in the care facility as she seeks empathic care from the staff. The Maternal also appears in many other aspects of Angelique's object-self relations and spiritual life.

Home as dwelling, inhabiting, welcoming hospitality, protective environment, nourishment, and origin

The thematization of the meanings of the home makes up a strong part of the bonding and caring experience that constitutes the Maternal Ground. Angelique describes her home in everyday terms, but it can be understood multidimensionally as a place of dwelling and inhabiting, a bastion of welcoming hospitality and a protective environment, a source of nourishment, and a point of origin. Angelique expresses jubilation upon the birth of her great-granddaughter and cherishes the opportunity to hold her, reflecting the meaning of the Maternal as dwelling and inhabiting:

> Yeah, my granddaughter had the baby, Madeline. ... Yes, the baby has been here. Everybody wanted to see the baby. Of course I hold the baby. Oh, yes. From the very day it was born, they gave the baby to me. So, Madeline is the baby's name. Marge and Magda. Because Marge is my child. ... and then Magda is Marge's daughter. Yes, and now Madeline is Magda's daughter. ... Madeline looked bigger today. And she's heavy. Yes, Magda is breastfeeding her.

Angelique expresses a Maternal, caring attitude toward her great-granddaughter, and shows openness and receptivity to her. For Angelique, this attitude of caring and receptivity in its meaning establishes a sense of the baby's belonging to the Maternal and to a community housed in the Maternal. Dwelling and inhabiting in the Maternal embrace are essential to the Maternal relation and the experience of being nurtured, starting in the womb. Angelique's descriptions of acts of Maternal care constitute forms of sociality or social cohesion that are transmitted from one generation to the next, and hold the family and community together.

The Maternal dimensions of dwelling and inhabiting in Angelique's experiences make possible the conditions for agency. The mother cradles the baby, creating the scaffolding for the developing young child's security and taking up of an agentic stance in the world in order to establish a sense of place, even amidst threats from the outside. This stance carries an attitude of meeting the world with openness and authority, as demonstrated below in Angelique's description of her early life experiences of inhabiting the Maternal region, when she learned to stand on her own facing the world:

> Yes, my grandmother took us to school. ... Everybody had to stay in this school because we had a disaster. ... The houses, there wasn't much anyway, but they blew down. I remember living through all of that. I remember the night of the hurricane. They put us in a trunk with a piece of board, and they sit us all there. Cover us up with a sheet under a tree. So. We were in between land and water. ... But it was bad and it was good. Taught us how to stand on our two feet.

For Angelique, these manifestations of the Maternal simultaneously provide protection from danger and create independence. The "standing on two feet" that Angelique describes is laden with significance. This upright posture points toward inhabiting, free agency, creativity, generativity, and expanding temporality and spatiality—all of which originate in the Maternal dwelling of nourishment, care, comfort, security, and well-being. This posture incubates agency, agentic processes, and action. It is an agentic stance, as it is always an intentionality, but in this case an empty intentionality through which Angelique seeks satisfaction of meaning through independence. It carries the potentiality for limitless subjective enactments and achievements in Angelique's future experience. In recalling past experiences from her early life and their core meanings of self-agency, Angelique thematizes the Maternal dimensions of the home and takes up an agentic stance in her current situation in the care facility.

Angelique's experience of the Maternal also exists in her having occupied the position of mother and in the agency she developed in the role of the person responsible for the care and raising of others. The birth of Angelique's great-granddaughter reminds Angelique of her own birthing experiences. She reflects on holding the baby in the womb, her experience of bathing pre-birth and her water breaking, the pain-free experience of the birth itself and bringing the baby home:

> The doctor told me I was going to have a baby. I had the baby. ... Yes, she was early. Oh, for me, it was lovely. I didn't have any pains. ... And when the water break, I tell my father-in-law to come take me to the hospital because my husband was going to work. ... When I went to the hospital, they took me upstairs and they gave me a bath, and he gave me a bell. Every time I get a pain, to ring the bell. So I never did get a pain. ... And I spent twelve days in the hospital... Twelve days with the baby. That's right. That's right, first experience in the hospital. Mm-hmm. It was lovely. To know you would bring home the baby. That was 55 years ago. I was 35. That was a very happy day, because I know it's not an easy thing, and some people have it so long. I think I was lucky. I gave God thanks.

Angelique's focus on the absence of pain in the birthing experience is striking. This pain-free state contrasts with the bodily and emotional pain she undergoes now in her frail state as she approaches the end of life. The Maternal womb—both the one she inhabited as a fetus and the one she provided to her own growing babies—is always the primordial first home, unreconstructed and uninterrupted, and one in which the Maternal amniotic fluid surrounds and protects the baby, providing unconditional, welcoming hospitality. In the care facility environment, Angelique yearns for Maternal care in her relationships with professional and family caregivers at the end of her life: she shows a desire to re-enact the security, nurturing, and happiness of this protected state. Angelique yearns for well-being, and relief from the burden of illness that weighs upon her in her frail, chronically ill, suffering condition. Implicit in Angelique's desire is the recognition that the well-being of the Maternal womb never can be achieved again in its pure, unconditional, and original state. The Maternal experienced amid frailty and serious illness in a care facility will always be a deficient mode of being because a need for relational empathic care in such circumstances never can be completely satisfied.

The home as place of origin—the horizon of experience in which retentions of past experiences from Angelique's birth have been sedimented and deposited—has multiple meanings for Angelique. The retained Maternal home stands in contrast to Angelique's experience of present frailty, illness, and dislocation at the end of her life in the care facility. But origin also has meaning in the sense of a futural horizon of experience. Angelique uses her projective capacities to imagine her continued connectedness with her roots and her timeless re-enactments of the security, comfort, and happiness of the Maternal dimensions of existence.

The varied meanings of home are intertwined and embedded within the Maternal. The home as well-being and happiness assumes initial form in the materiality of the mother's milk and body as home, and evolves as a place of dwelling—as welcoming hospitality and protective environment, as source of nourishment and development, as the ground of an agentic stance, and as origin.

Dynamic opposition between the home and the realm of suffering

Angelique's story shows a dynamic opposition between the home as a fundamentally positive, supporting constituent of the Maternal Ground and as a realm of suffering and impoverishment located outside the Maternal and experienced as alien, even potentially threatening. Angelique's earlier description of surviving the hurricane, with a makeshift shelter and a feeling that the permanence of home is illusory, implicitly captures this tension and this realm in her early life in broad terms:

> Where I live in the islands … since the volcano came, Americans split our packages. When I say "packages"—our land. And they gave half to the people that was coming to America, and the other half is for us. So they just take ours, and built a bridge or something. … We belong to the English country.

Angelique's description suggests that the meaning of what exists outside the Maternal dwelling involves a threat—an appropriation of something that did not belong to the usurpers, as well as a displacement. The home and the realm of suffering and impoverishment outside the home have a shifting temporality and spatiality as Angelique negotiates her changing life-world.

Desire for self-actualizing at the end of life

The persistence of desire in lived experiences of suffering is essential to the Maternal. Desire is an emotionally rich intentionality and a temporal movement toward something else—becoming. Angelique strives for well-being, sociality, relational care, intimacy, generativity, and fidelity.

The Maternal relation and caring experience form the ground for Angelique's growth, development, and well-being at the end of life. Fidelity as a constituent of Maternal well-being figures prominently as a meaning that Angelique values in her life-world. For Angelique, fidelity means constancy and faith—in her relationships with family members and with God, in her agentic and vocational pursuits, and in her future. In Angelique's descriptions, retentions of the Maternal lay the foundation for core meanings of loving care, empathy, fidelity, and faith that Angelique desires in her interpersonal relationships with others. The Maternal nourishment of the child Angelique's ego prepares her for living in and enjoying the world as both a child and an adult. Angelique's early experiences of receiving profound love and care in relationships with her mother, grandmother, and great-grandmother create a personal history that shapes her later experiences, including her desires for the constancy and fidelity of relational, empathic care at the end of life.

Angelique recalls going to church with her mother and learning how to pray. She reflects on her mother's productive work in weeding the garden and raising cotton, work that had a generative capacity for Angelique even in their poverty. She experiences these forms of care as nourishing and growth-producing, and they become the ground of her relationship as an adult with her own children, whom she cares for in the same loving way with generative capacities:

> I have a lot of faith in God. Faith is very important to me. Very much so. My mother took us to church. She was very poor. … I was not born in America. I was born in the islands. … I was twenty-nine when I came here. Very poor. But we make it. We made the bad with the good, mixed the bad with the good. My mother did outside work, like weed the garden, weed the cotton, that kind of work. …
>
> Of course, she taught me how to pray and to have faith. … I brought my children up the same way. They had two dresses, one for school and one for church. Until finally that I got a machine and I made their dresses. Right now, I'm making little ones for that lady, I mean the baby. Mm-hmm. I made all my clothes, for my daughters. … I'm still—if my hands would give me a break, I still will make dresses. That's what my life is.

Angelique's position as a mother who nurtured and raised her children is essential to her meanings of the Maternal Ground. Her positions as caregiver and care-recipient play a key role in the satisfaction of higher-order needs for fulfillment of intentionalities. Both the ground of obligation for Angelique as an "I," and her responsibility to others, spring from and constitute the Maternal.

Maternal as Moral Agency and Community

In recalling and bringing to bear past experiences of the Maternal dimensions of existence, Angelique identifies the ethical dimensions and moral responsibilities in her situated relationships with others and place in communities. She speaks of "doing the best you know how" in her enactments and life's work. Angelique makes this kind of moral claim about the nature of her ethical relationship and moral responsibility to her significant others—her spouse and children in particular, but also her brother and her aunt:

> I would go visit Auntie … I go up. I comb her hair. I bathe her according to when she bathed last. Yes, I would take care of her. Bring her special food. … I used to do that for my aunt. Cook and take the food to her. For her. Give her a bath. Comb her hair. Right, take care of her like a mother would take care of a baby. Right. And I am, was, expecting my children to do the same thing.

In reflecting on her own end-of-life wishes, Angelique remembers the role she played in her brother's end-of-life planning and at the moment of his death in a poetic and uniquely cultural description of her presence and fidelity:

> I had a brother and he died. He said to me, "Angelique, don't—I don't want to be questioned by the doctors." At that time, they didn't have this here yet [a DNR order]. So I told him, "Yes, I understand." He tell me, "Yes." And when he died, I didn't have a problem. I was with him when he died. Foot-to-foot. And everything went on. That's the last that you are doing for them. Yes, I remember that experience with my brother.

Angelique experiences herself as an agent and a member of a moral community. She desires fidelity in her relationships with others, and in her relationships with her children, the same fidelity that she values in her relationship with God, and that orientation reveals itself in her descriptions of her faith and spirituality.

Conclusion

Angelique's testimony provides an in-depth portrait of suffering and its relationship to human development over the life course. First and foremost, suffering is part of the human condition and has its own intentional structure, with origins in the earliest stages of human development and in the Maternal dimensions of existence, and is not reducible to medical diagnoses or pathologizing. The suffering of seriously ill elderly persons, such as Angelique, and their agentic responses to illness burden are revealed as surpassing the limitations of end-of-life illness, and ultimately concerning the tasks, hopes, and liberating dreams of living as a free agent in a fundamentally social world.

Phenomenologist John Drummond (2008a) helps to illuminate the paradox of suffering and its intentional structure in explaining that moral phenomenology involves three different meanings of consciousness:

> (1) consciousness as the interweavings of experience that make up a unified stream of experience, that make up, if you will, the first person or subject; (2) consciousness as self-awareness, the intransitive, phenomenal consciousness with which the narrow conception of phenomenology is concerned; and (3) consciousness as the intentional directedness to objects other than the experiencing self, the transitive consciousness understood as taking an object.
>
> (p. 36)

It is in the third type of consciousness enumerated by Drummond that we can locate the suffering and strivings of Angelique, as well as the elders in the chapter narratives that follow.

This reframing of suffering does not diminish, but rather strengthens, the call for non-abandonment and empathic care responses to suffering persons. Attunement to more humanistic, person-centered practice with seriously ill persons in light of their lived experiences of suffering help minimize the impact of social structures and conditions that may impede access to good medical care and symptom management. In Chapter 7, examples of such care among seriously ill elders, who turn to institutions for the empathic, Maternal care, food and security they have been unable to find in the harsh outside world, are described. An ethic of care that is built upon empathic relationships, shows respect for the dignity of the person, empowers the person to recover lost agency in emotional attachments and re-enactments of the lived past even in the presence of dementias, heightens the person's sense of well-being, and provides critical support to seriously ill persons.

3 The Social Ecology of Suffering and Chronic Pain in Serious Illness
Traumatic Losses of Maternal Foundations

In his differentiations of life forms from symbols and concepts, Alfred Schütz posited that there are layers of experience that are not accessible to language, but there are certain forms of non-verbal communication that do reach these deeper layers of experience (Barber, 2013). Experiences of suffering, as well as chronic pain, among seriously ill older adults may fall within those realms of experience that cannot be easily translated into ordinary language precisely because they draw on implicit, unknown, or concealed horizons. In this chapter, I describe traumatic losses Angelique experiences in making the transition to life in the care facility, and the pairing of the suffering of Angelique's life-world existence with multiple transcendent realities afforded through the symbolic presence of the Maternal—and what it symbolizes—in the everyday world.

Central Temporal Moment: Vortex of Pain and Suffering

The social ecology of pain and suffering in serious illness, is informed by the narrative of Angelique and her chronic care experiences. Systems of pain and suffering were salient in Angelique's life-world. After being admitted to the care facility, Angelique was thrown into a vortex of bodily pain and emotional turmoil from which she struggled to extricate herself.

Dislocation and loss of home

Angelique's move to the care facility had meanings of appropriation and displacement for her. Her home was taken from her, and she was displaced from her place of dwelling. This loss of her sense of place and of belonging to a life-world that she knew were forms of pain and suffering for her in her increasingly frail and dependent state.

The realm in which Angelique became situated in the care facility, which she perceived as neither a place of dwelling nor a Maternal home, had certain descriptive characteristics that stood in opposition to the home, an opposition between the lost Maternal home and the mode of being in the realm of suffering outside the home. In this second temporal moment of Angelique's development, these are anti-Maternal. This opposition was one between love of life, thriving, enjoyment, and development versus impoverishment, decline, and threat. Angelique described having no money, no help, no companionship, no emotional support or satisfaction, no place to go in this realm:

> So… yet sometimes I feel that that is better for me than to be knocking around at people's house. So, that's the way it goes. But when talking about the help, you asked me—I don't get no help. M. [the hospice aide] only makes up the bed. Not sweeping.
>
> I think they don't—I got to have everything paid for. I really didn't hide— she [Angelique's daughter] didn't hide anything, and I say anything. She tell them [the care facility] what is what—so that's how it go. But sometimes I just cry because living in a—what made me get angry more is when I come home of an evening from—what they call that place? From therapy in the building. We go to class. I feel so lonesome and upset.
>
> I want to say a few words to L, my daughter.
>
> I have to do something. Because I have this—I don't have any money. What I had I give it to my daughter. Know you can't have the house and come to the care facility. Yes. So she's living in the house. House coming down that hill there. It's a house. That's where I always live in. No, I didn't raise my children there, because I moved over here lately. So. But Marge moved way up there. But she's going to have a baby. Marge's daughter, Magda, is having the baby. I was living there before I came here.
>
> Yes, that was a special place to me; that was a special place.
>
> If I could get out, I would get out. I can't go back there because, you know, if you have a house you have to pay so much more for it.
>
> I haven't been home in a long time. Home worries me a lot. Worries me. What worries me is that I don't have a place where I could go and come home by myself.

The realm in which Angelique was situated in the care facility had core meanings of suffering for her. Phenomenologically, the care facility did not even have the meaning of a place for Angelique. She described her liminality: "I don't have a place where I could go and come home by myself." What she had lost was a home that brought forth life, a special place, as she described it, that continued to tease recollections of her past experiences of the security, comfort, and uninterrupted happiness of dwelling in the security of Maternal arms. She had to make a tradeoff in giving up her house in order to come to the care facility. She suggested that maybe things could be worse, but the bargain she made involved surrendering her economic and social independence.

Angelique perceived herself as reduced to a state of dependency on an aide who performed certain perfunctory tasks, but was not someone to whom she could turn for the kind of empathic care she was seeking. She was caught in a life-world transition from a known world to one completely unknown and uncertain. She acknowledged feeling confused and disoriented at times—but beyond simple loss of memory or failure to recall where she physically resided. Her disorientation extended to her social, moral, and spiritual displacement as a relational other—a person who had been connected to her meaningful loved ones, from whom she now felt alienated. In making this transition, she longed for the care that she once drew upon while living within the Maternal dimensions of existence. The experience of the home was essentially an other-oriented and relational experience. Angelique's displacement from her home severed her connectedness with her place of dwelling and her world, and the meanings that they had for her and her relational others. This sense of homelessness, isolation, and lack of a vital and animating connection to home and others was a source of great suffering for her. Her expressions of being lonesome were expressions of a desire for social connection and an awareness that her current mode of being was deficient. This motivated a desire for self-development, self-efficacy, and agency.

The home and the realm of suffering and impoverishment that exist outside the home took on a shifting temporality and spatiality as Angelique negotiated her changing life-world. The boundaries of these systems were fluid and constantly in flux. Angelique's transition to the care facility was characterized by the dominance in her life-world of the realm outside the home that continued while she experienced the loss of the Maternal Foundations and a supportive home, the loss of sociality and relationality, and the loss of agency as significant sources of personal and existential suffering. However, the recovery of agency and a Maternal homecoming were accompanied by an expansion of spatiality, temporality, spirituality, and existential and spiritual transcendence, effectively diminishing the influence of the anti-maternal realm.

Affective desire

Angelique communicated a desire for the meanings of the Maternal dimensions of existence, a desire that has affective dimensions and a desire that is not yet fulfilled:

> I feel all right, but people have been giving me a lot of trouble… problems. I can't reach my mother, I can't reach my sisters, so I am just in the lonesome path.

Angelique feels alone in her new environment and emotional anguish in response to these feelings. Regular visits from family members did not allay her overwhelming sense of isolation and separation from her loved ones and her home. She spoke of living with her family for all those years and conveyed a strong conception of being rooted. Her move to the care facility decentered and de-anchored her and left her feeling homeless. Family visits did not substitute for the home she had lost. Angelique expressed an intense desire for social engagement, to be with her family and to have deep relational connections with family members. Her consciousness was directed toward these goals, and her emotional responses to the loss of these relational connections disclosed their deep relational meaning to her:

Only that sometime I am very lonesome. I am lonesome at the shelter, at the home. I am lonesome now. Sometimes I feel I want to see them [family]… and it's not so pleasant. While I am here, I would like to see them. I see them too, you know. I see them… it's not to say I don't see them. Yesterday they were here. That's like when Sunday come—they take off a Sunday and come to see me. So I wouldn't say that they don't bother with me; that would be a lie. But maybe being living with them all the years—that's what made me feel that way. So when they are not here, I am missing them. Of course, I miss them badly. I wish they were here. That's what I am talking about. Sometimes I am all right, but sometimes I just miss them a lot. And that is why I am here. No, I don't talk to the social worker or the doctor.

In addition to Angelique's loneliness and clear desire for social connection, Angelique uses the word "shelter" to describe the care facility. The meaning of the care facility to Angelique was akin to a place of last resort for the homeless, the forsaken, the abandoned.

While Angelique expressed a general sense of well-being, or feeling "all right" that survived through these suffering experiences in the care facility, it was clear that she felt abandoned by her caregivers, and that she was not receiving the kind of support she felt she needed to cope with the trauma of dislocation that she was experiencing.

Angelique suffered the loss of sociality, relationality, and home as well as the concomitant loss of autonomy, control, and agency. The contours of the social ecology of suffering and end-of-life decision making of a frail elderly woman making transitions to living the last months of her life in a care facility emerge from the narrative. Angelique felt homeless, in an environment she distrusted, and even though she saw her family, she experienced a feeling of being banished to a shrunken space that was not shared with or by them. They had to some extent become outsiders, remote and unavailable to her in her new life-world. Angelique turned to invoking the Maternal, yet the Maternal relational system she sought and its essential constituents of the welcoming home and compassionate care were not yet accessible to her. While Angelique made this migration from her old home to a reconstructed home, from the life she had given up to the possibilities of a new life, the space she occupied was barren and desolate, offering her little in the way of nurture, comfort, or care. She desired relief from her suffering in a place of rescue where she could go to find rest:

All I am interested in is to find a nice place where I can come in and sit down and relax and rest. That's my aim. Rest is here. I'm here. And right now, I'm thinking of something that I want. I want to leave here. No. Get a different place. Mm-hmm. I'm hoping. And praying. Yeah, and that's what I am asking God for.

Angelique desired the practical concerns of living, such as walking. Angelique had lost the ability to walk, and this was a form of both pain and suffering for her.

The loss of ambulation was a concomitant loss of agency for Angelique. This loss was related to the decline in health and increasing disabilities resulting from her illness process. Angelique's desire for physical therapy involved both a reconstitution of nurturing material support on the social level as well as active efforts on her part to resume her agency. Her desire was pervasive throughout the narrative data, especially in her overriding concern that she was not receiving the physical therapy services that would enable her to achieve mobility or maintain the level of functioning that she would like:

> I thought by now I would get my health—my foot better. My foot cannot be turned. Do you understand? My knee hurts, not in pain while I am sitting or when I am sleeping. But I have pain, especially when I get up.
>
> I try to get up—it is so hard. Anyway, I used to get PT a long time and they stopped it and I don't know why because I cannot walk. I don't know why the PT stopped, because they don't tell me anything. No, they didn't tell me why it stopped. Yes, I am unhappy that the PT stopped, for the reason that I am looking forward to walk again. So. No, I am not able to walk. Right, I spend most of my time in the wheelchair. See, I can't get up as I should.

Angelique desires to walk, but also desires expanding spatiality and temporality, health and improved functioning, and overall well-being. Angelique's desires and agency arose from her experience of pain, both the bodily pain she experienced in her knee when she tried to get up and the emotional response of unhappiness that was part of her pain experience. These desires acted as powerful motivators for self-agency.

Pain as a social and relational system

The experience of pain grew out of Angelique's end-of-life illnesses and frailty. She first became aware of her frailty when she broke her hand and could no longer remain in her home. She consented to a transfer to the care facility that was arranged by her family. As Angelique became situated in the care facility, her frailty became apparent to her in the form of limitations on her activities of daily living. She described these limitations: she could not hold anything in her hands, she could not walk, she could not stand, she had no physical energy. She felt that the weakness in her lower extremities had gotten worse since she had come to the facility, increasingly so with the discontinuation of her physical therapy. Her bodily weakness and inability to do things on her own were the core meanings of frailty for Angelique, and she perceived that as a result of her frailty she was dependent on others to help her, especially because her hands were so disabled.

Angelique demonstrated her dependency and current wishes to be cared for, washed, and soothed in a relationally empathic and intimate way reminiscent of an infant in a syncretic state:

> Yeah, I'm sore now. Did I tell them? I think, yes. Because I asked them for A+D. They gave [it to] the girl who is going to take care of me. Yes. And I tell the girl, "Please rub my back [sic.] hind with that A+D ointment." Because it is very cool. Yes, they use it for the babies. Yes, she put it on me. Yes, it felt better. Well, when you have that on, it stops hurting you or burning you. Uh-huh, the burning stops. But it's not easy. Sometimes you put your confidence in them [the aide or nurse]. It doesn't work, you know. So what are you going to do? You can't do anything. You can't fight them.

Angelique was not able to relieve her pain and suffering on her own—she felt helpless. She was dependent on others to hold and rescue her. Her agency was exercised as an appeal to the caregiver. The losses of other types of agency and empowerment in this situation were a significant part of Angelique's suffering. She was not only experiencing pain and burning, but she could not eliminate these feelings herself as she might have at other times in her life course, and as she did when she gave birth to her daughter.

Angelique disclosed that she knew her medical diagnoses and she named them as "Parkinson's and blood pressure." She made the connection that she was taking medications to treat these medical problems. However, it was the experience of physical limitations in the use of her hands and her lower extremities, her loss of weight, loss of functioning, frailty, and the concomitant social and emotional limitations that created for her an inexorable movement toward the experience of end-of-life illness. Angelique's experience of illness was not medical alone, but social and existential, founded on lived burdens of pain and suffering imposed on her by her life-limiting and life-threatening conditions.

Angelique's experience of pain had subjective and existential dimensions:

> Look here, look at that foot here. It's sore and that's why I can't walk. I have a toothache. I have a lot of things… sometimes I just sit down and cry and say I should've… if I knew that I was going to fall into hands like this, I would've stayed there—there and that will be it—cause that's where I was born.
>
> Yesterday morning, yesterday night and morning, this hand hurt me. Both. Two of them. But this right one here. Yes, they're both hurting me. Yes. But you feel how tight they [hands] are? I have to—yesterday morning, not this morning, yesterday morning—they hurt me so bad until I wanted to cry out.
>
> But if you even cry out, they don't bother with you. Even if you cry out, they don't want to bother with you. I was in such pain. But God is good. No pain medication. They say they give me Tylenol. It didn't help. But I'm not—I can't take it that time because I'm not supposed to get up out of bed. And they tell me, they're saying that they're doing their best. The workers don't come out.

Angelique spoke explicitly about her experiences of pain. Her pain is multidimensional—physical, emotional, social, relational, spiritual, and cultural. These dimensions of Angelique's pain are not segregated, but primal moments that are a unitary experience. Angelique's frailty, physical limitations, and loss of functioning underlay her experience of pain. She had a palpable emotional response to her bodily pain and values it negatively. The pain was bad, intolerable, and imposed a heavy burden on her. Angelique displayed a strong emotional response to her pain, and a desire to return to her place of origin, the Maternal home. She experienced pain in her hands, in her foot, in her toes, in her knee, in her tooth, and in her intimate parts from improper toileting and from being confined to a wheelchair for long hours. But even while Angelique was in pain, she spoke of God's goodness. She described her experience of being in pain (the bad) and of transcending her pain (being in the presence of God) at the same time.

Angelique's pain management affected her pain trajectory. Some of the forms of pain that Angelique experienced were treated with medication, others were not. There were times when Angelique felt that her pain was untreated or undertreated, as in the example when she reported persistent pain in her hands. The intolerable pain that she underwent led to suffering. Angelique's testimony shows the very strong social and relational dimensions of pain experiences: the meaning of the pain experiences in the context of Angelique's social context, loss of Maternal Foundations, immersion in an alienating and unwelcoming environment, and as shrunken spatiality and temporality in her relations with family members and care facility staff.

In summary, Angelique's pain originated with a sensory, bodily experience to which she had both a bodily response and an emotional response. Her pain demanded a care response. The nature of the care response affected and influenced the course of Angelique's pain experience and her emotional response. If her pain was appropriately managed, she would experience less emotional arousal. However, if her pain was not appropriately managed, as she expressed in the foregoing example, her feelings of anxiety and frustration, and her perception of having diminished self-efficacy might contribute to an escalation of her pain and her developing or cultivated emotional response to experience of pain. Pain is a social developmental and relational system involving dialectical process interactions with the self and others that change over time. To Angelique, the occurrence of pain in the presence of the infinite goodness of God was an example of such dialectical movements. Angelique's limitations and experiences of pain did not interfere with her development, growth, and self-actualization at the end of life. Pain therefore has structural, social, developmental, and process dimensions, and cannot be reduced to sensory data or a medical outcome.

Traumatic suffering and its social developmental context

Angelique's persistent and untreated or undertreated pain led to her experience of suffering. She also experienced suffering that was not directly a consequence of her pain. This individual psychological structure is dominated by Angelique's suffering experience. Multiple sources of Angelique's suffering experiences temporally and spatially create the horizon structure of her dislocation, displacement, and alienation that surpasses her end-of-life illness and ultimately concerns her living. The depth and breadth of Angelique's malaise and misery are captured best in an episode about an experience involving what she called a "chicken head." This experience disclosed the nature of suffering not only as a thing that is experienced, but also as a temporal, social, and developmental event. The description also revealed Angelique's emotional state in response to her suffering experience in the care facility and the values she attached to her experience through a consciousness of suffering. As she expanded her consciousness of suffering, she expanded her consciousness of the possibility of detaching herself from suffering through spiritual movement and transcendence. This is the nexus of suffering and the Maternal: the givenness and affordances of the Maternal provide the conditions of possibility for detaching oneself from suffering, the conditions for the possibility of agency, sociality, and spirituality.

Angelique described receiving a plate from the care facility staff during the lunchtime meal with the other residents, and described further seeing the "head of a chicken" on the plate.[1] She experienced the "chicken head" as a trauma that shocked her sensibilities, assaulted her dignity, and relegated her to a marginalized position in the care facility community as someone who was stigmatized. Angelique revealed that she had never seen the head of a chicken before, or purchased or cooked a chicken with a head on it. She stated that she was the only resident who received a plate with a chicken head on it:

> They cook one day, and what they did, they put a chicken head in my plate. Uh-huh. I mean, that's a chicken head. I mean, that's a chicken head—not turkey. I mean, that's a chicken head. And one of the girls said, "She [Angelique] could have said she didn't like chicken head." Why a chicken head have to be in my plate? You know? That's all what they're doing to me.
>
> I don't know where they got it. They cooked lunch and a chicken head. I have never cooked a chicken head yet in my life. An actual head of a chicken. Because you buy the chicken, they don't give you the head.
>
> Yes. Recently, two weeks ago now. Terrible.
>
> I hollered, "So why you all have to put a chicken head in my plate? I don't cook chicken head for myself." So one of the other aides or servants said, "She [Angelique] could have said she no like chicken head." Why should I have to say so? You cook a chicken, you put that chicken on the [plate], because chicken head, you don't really see. I was going to tell her, because I don't get to tell her. Now, my nurse gets angry at me because I said, "The food is cold. I don't want cold food. I eat food, but not cold like this." But I'm eating up, too.
>
> I'm eating up all these things. And it's not the best thing for me because I said, "What the hell you all think I am? Really, I have to tell you what I say?"
>
> Yeah, that was the worst thing that ever happened to me here. Of course. It was very upsetting.
>
> Who did I tell? I don't even remember. Yes, the other residents see it, because I held it out. Some of them, they laughed. Mm-hmm [they laughed].

Angelique's interpretation of this experience has great significance in the overall context of her suffering, her life course trajectory, and her end of life. Angelique self-identified as an oppressed person, a sufferer, and someone who was branded as a sufferer. The magnitude of this self-identification reached far beyond the meaning of her end-of-life illnesses. It went back to her origin and experiences growing up poor in marginalized communities, losing her two husbands to cancer and fighting to sustain a family as a single mother, and now living in a care facility in which, as an indigent, dually-eligible care facility resident, she continued to be a member of a marginalized community with limited access to resources. She was a displaced person. Her immersion in this experience of displacement was part of her self-identification with the Maternal dimensions of existence and past retentions of being in a syncretic, holding environment.

Angelique experienced the marginalized position she felt she was in as in some way a fall from a height, accompanied by feelings of loss of dignity, loss of self, loss of identity, loss of humanity, and voicelessness. Despite these assaults on her dignity and humanity, Angelique drew upon her personal resources and other past experiences of the Maternal dimensions of existence in which she was first acculturated to form an upright posture and an agentic stance of resistance against oppression in the care facility.

What made this experience particularly horrible for Angelique was that she was unable to tell anyone about it. She felt she had no voice and could not be heard. Communication is founded upon relationality. Angelique's removal from relational intimacy with family members, caregivers, and others in the care facility community severely constrained her opportunities for conversation and meaningful communication. She could not reach any member of her family to let them know what had happened to her; she could not communicate with the staff whom she felt had witnessed her affliction with little show of empathy; similarly, she could not turn to the other residents, as they showed no understanding of her situation. Therefore, she perceived that she was left to suffer in her misery alone and in isolation, with no empathic care or relief from her suffering.

Even though this episode did not happen, Angelique experienced it in revealing ways. Angelique made reference to how hard things were for her. She said this in a couple of different ways to describe the extent of her burden. She described an experience of having a staff person dig her nails into her flesh when she was being showered. Her burden was extraordinary, approaching a level of dehumanization, and she suggested that she experienced apprehension about whether she would be able to sustain this kind of burden indefinitely. She spoke of having to resort to "going to court" to get relief from this intolerable suffering. The core meaning of suffering for Angelique in this trauma was that every aspect of her experience, her perceptions of self-efficacy, and her agentic capacity to respond to the experience in the present were threatened. Her affliction, accumulation of burden, and partially disabled agency also threatened her futural horizon of experience.

This "chicken head" episode is illustrative of the type of traumatic suffering Angelique experienced, involving loss of Maternal Foundations on which her existence rested. These foundations had deep social and cultural significance for her. The constituents of Angelique's traumatic suffering were losses of dignity, self, humanity, role, autonomy, self-efficacy, and fulfilling agency; losses of the welcoming home, boundaries, and family and social structures; losses of sociality and community, relational discontinuity with family members, and the absence of meaningful relationships with professional caregivers; accumulation of burden, and a pervasive sense of affliction in her end-of-life illness from which there was no relief or rescue.

Conclusion

The multiple losses of Maternal Foundations and loss of agency experienced by Angelique were found to be invariant in the structure of suffering at high level generality in the main study and the follow-up study across all the study participants, and even beyond them, among seriously ill older adults in care facility environments. Through Angelique's testimony, phenomenological methods gave access to elders' meanings of their temporal suffering experience and its origins in human development that connect back to primordial Maternal dimensions of existence. In the chapters that follow, I explore these meanings further, as well as an agentic, life-affirming, and empathic care-seeking drive and type of well-being among elderly women and men.

Note

1   The non-veridicality of this "chicken head" episode was established. The use of bracketing assures that the non-veridicality has no bearing on understanding the meaning of the experience for Angelique.

4 Suffering and Care-Seeking as Moral Experience

Movement Toward Self-Actualization and Spiritual Well-Being

Angelique's taking up of decisions near the end of life are part of her movement toward self-actualization and well-being, and are constitutively moral experiences. Angelique's Maternal homecoming involves her re-enactment and achievement of an overall sense of spiritual well-being and fidelity to her intentions at the end of her life. This sense of spiritual well-being is co-occurrent with her experiences of pain and suffering as well as movements toward self-actualization and existential transcendence, and is a fulfillment of the meaning of Angelique's intention to return home and be at rest. An important finding of this research is the duality of lived experience and the enormous capacities of the frail elderly person to hold conflicting and contradictory experiences in her spatio-temporal horizon. These conflicting and contradictory dimensions of lived experience are shifting, sometimes in small ebbs and flows and sometimes like tsunamis, as in her "chicken head" trauma—disrupting her life-world and opening up opportunities for transformation and change. Angelique's spiritual life and the Maternal Ground upon which it rests help to nurture and sustain her, and offer her hope for a future even as she lives with an illness burden of life-limiting and life-threatening multi-morbidity through these ebbs and flows.

Elder decision making, relational end-of-life planning, and communication

Angelique is engaged in end-of-life planning and decision-making processes, and demonstrates her openness to such processes. For Angelique, decision making is a process that is ongoing, multidimensional, and evolutionary. It includes decisions about health care treatment and her person-centered care needs, such as whom she trusts to make decisions for her when she no longer has capacity, and future planning decisions. Finally, it is a process that is both social—because it involves social systems in which Angelique is embedded such as those of family and of provider—and self-directed, and driven by self-agency. Decision making is characterized by a high degree of self-control, self-efficacy, and agency, and involves cognitive, affective, social, and cultural dimensions.

Angelique has a Do Not Resuscitate Order and a health care proxy. Her engagement in forms of end-of-life planning is a decision process in itself and involves desire and agency. But what distinguishes the end-of-life planning decision process from everyday decision making is the goal toward which Angelique's agency is directed—her own end of life. She embraces the fact that the horizon structure of suffering in end-of-life decision making has an end of life in the futural horizon about which she can make decisions in the present. One of those decisions is the appointment of her daughter as the person she trusts to make decisions for her and "take charge" of everything. She has also had meaningful conversations with her daughter about end-of-life care options—such as feedings tubes and burial arrangements. The centrality of communication to Angelique's relational meanings and conversations is salient in the end-of-life planning discussions she has with her daughter. The choices and decisions Angelique makes depend on her being able to communicate those choices and decisions effectively to her daughter, whom she has appointed to be her health care agent and to act for her when she no longer has capacity. The trust she has in her daughter and their relational intimacy found the type of communication they have—the good conversations. Therefore, there is valuing involved in decision making. Angelique attaches value attributes to her decision process and her decision outcomes.

She describes the experiences she lived through with her two husbands, both of whom died of cancer, and her brother, to whom she remained faithful, "foot-to-foot," until his death. In recalling these past experiences, she expresses her own end-of-life wishes about her future care planning in her current situation in the care facility, and about the kind of care, attention, and fidelity she expects from her relational caregivers. In discussing her burial arrangements, she freely discusses the hymns she has thought about. She shows no discomfort in having these discussions about her end of life or engaging in the complex thought and decision-making processes involved in forgoing treatment.

Angelique appeals to her caregiver to rub ointment on her perineum to relieve the soreness and burning she is experiencing. This is an example of Angelique's coping with her suffering condition through decision making about her care—a manifestation of her agency. Her decision has the meaning of an attempt to restore the Maternal relation and, through it, embodied comfort and security, in order to eliminate the detrimental aspects of her world.

The decision to forgo cardiopulmonary resuscitation in the event of cardiac arrest reflects the agentic processes at work in Angelique's end-of-life decision making. Forgoing treatment is a complex decision process because it involves weighing alternative treatments and their risks, benefits, and burdens, deliberating about the alternatives, and making a judgment. In this process, Angelique's end of life becomes thematic for her. She evaluates the burden to herself of life-sustaining treatment that is likely to heighten her suffering and be a burden to relational others. She also evaluates the alternative of refusing life-sustaining treatment, choosing to have a natural death that is unassisted by medical technology, which may assure her relief from the burden of suffering in a futural horizon. She testifies that she does not wish to be a burden to her family. The concept of burden complicates the end-of-life decision-making process with social and relational dimensions.

Relationships with health care professionals

Angelique's relationships with her health care professionals and direct care staff are part of her situatedness in the care facility community and environment, and are part of the social context of decision making. Overall, Angelique does not have well-developed relationships with the professionals or staff of the care facility. This is particularly devastating for her given the relational discontinuity she has with family members. She does not express confidence in her doctor, psychologist, or spiritual care professionals, and cites infrequent conversations with her social worker. The relational problems that she has with staff weaken communication about Angelique's goals of care.

Types of health care decisions

There are three types of treatment decisions in which Angelique is involved in the care facility: i) decisions that involve routine health or custodial care; ii) decisions that involve functioning such as physical therapy services; and iii) major decisions such as changes in the goals of care and alignment of treatment with such goals that are related to the trajectory of Angelique's illnesses.

Angelique's concern with the various types of health care decisions in the care facility relate to her sense of health and well-being. One type of decision about self-care involves everyday choices and deliberations, such as seeking medication for pain or soothing ointment for raw and irritated tissue. While certain areas of everyday decision making can be viewed as routine, as they involve regular care needs, the elder's experience of the illness or the care need cannot be described as routine. Angelique experiences chronic pain in her knees and in her hands. Her pain level is assessed as "none" or "controlled" in her medical records, but differs from her communication of her pain experience. There is a moral claim for relief of pain made by Angelique. Independent of the objective intensity and quality of the pain, assessment and treatment of any pain are not routine. Abandonment of the elder in a state of pain heightens the person's pain and leads to suffering.

Other types of routine decisions in which Angelique is involved are decisions that affect her functional level. She experiences perhaps the most anguish about her health care that relates to her functional decline in ambulation. This concern is directly related to the discontinuation of physical therapy by the care facility staff during the period documented in the medical record prior to discharge from hospice.

In light of Angelique's burning desire to walk and to achieve mobility, she greets this discontinuation of physical therapy services with terrible frustration and rage. She also expresses persistent unhappiness that she was not made a part of the care planning conversations that led to this decision to terminate the physical therapy service. This issue has meaning for Angelique in terms of communication and the decision-making process. She feels that not only has she suffered relational losses, but also that these losses have been compounded by communication failures. She experiences a connection between interpersonal relations and communication. For Angelique, relationality founds communication in the

Maternal system and in the systems the Maternal founds; weak interpersonal relationships appear to limit effective communication between Angelique and her health care professionals.

In this context, decision making and its constitutive processes of deliberation and practical evaluation are expressions of agency. Angelique draws upon this powerful sense of agency in the process of decision making involving her health care professionals at the care facility, which she experiences as giving her very little voice in making decisions about her care.

A major health care decision for Angelique in the care facility is both the admission to and discharge from hospice. Angelique communicates a weak sense of agency about the decision to be enrolled in hospice, and about the decision to be discharged when she begins to flourish and is no longer eligible for hospice services. This means that she does not seem to fully comprehend the nature of the decisions made and her "authoring" of the decision process. She suggests that she did not participate in the decision process. The decision was presented to her as a factual state of affairs. However, she is by no means passive or non-agentic. She does share that she was told post-facto that she was on hospice and, after the adjustment, has tried to adapt to this change and accept that this is probably the best path for her at this stage of her illness. Throughout her hospice stay, however, she has struggled to make herself a decision-maker by reflecting on and challenging her post-decision state of affairs. Angelique questions why she is not receiving physical therapy services, and protests the inability of her hospice aide to assist her with walking. She has a passionate desire to walk and will not allow her desire to be extinguished by her enrollment in hospice. She persists in questioning why she is not receiving physical therapy services and why she did not participate more fully in the decision-making process for her to go on hospice. Angelique does not understand the role of the hospice aide, and experiences a high level of frustration that her intention to achieve mobility is not enabled. Communication emerges as a theme in her testimony with respect to this major decision:

> Excuse me a little… what's her name now, M—[the hospice aide]? So… that's—I told M—to let—M—is the girl that you all paid to sit here with me, right? M—sits with me. Oh, you didn't know about it, too? Well, I don't know.
>
> They didn't put it through me. It was after they finished, they tell me that they pick a girl to come in early in the morning and sit with me and if I want anything upstairs, she [M—] could do that.
>
> "Who is that?" No, no, no. M—alone. She alone. . . No, this girl here—this M—here. She's supposed to… I wasn't… That's my daughter and… My daughter was involved in the decision. I think so. Because I wasn't there. No.
>
> So the details I don't know, but she's supposed to come in and, when I left, she's supposed to make the bed and straighten up the room. So, that's as much as I could tell you about it. So… I haven't spoken to anybody. Anyway.
>
> No, I only heard the name "hospice." But not anybody tell me anything. Because I was even kind of scared to hear the word hospice and—but now I

am getting accustomed here… and don't tell anybody that I am around hospice. They say, "Mammy, that's the best—that's the best for you because you know we don't have anybody at home to stay with you and I am afraid when you cook, you might leave the gas on." So that's why I am here. So that's my story.

To be assessed for and enrolled in hospice care is a major treatment decision for Angelique, but she makes very clear that this was a decision process from which she felt distanced and excluded. She describes being told of the decision after she was enrolled in hospice when she was introduced to M, her hospice aide.

Angelique understands what hospice is and, although she confesses that at first it frightened her, she believes that she could have benefited from the care once she understood it. But M, the hospice aide, did not meet her expectations in terms of care. Angelique had a strong desire to walk, and expected that the hospice aide would assist her in achieving her goals to improve her functioning. Angelique experienced high levels of distress in connection with the misalignment between her goals of care and the care she was receiving. Angelique accepted hospice to the extent that it meant she was becoming increasingly frail and approaching the end of life, but she did not understand that she would no longer have access to physical therapy services or would face a significant decline in functioning. Moreover, when hospice care was discontinued, Angelique felt that she was not informed of the change in goals of care and she was not able to exercise self-determination or control. This surrendering of autonomy in decision making and the diminution of perceptions of self-efficacy are forms of suffering for Angelique in the care facility environment.

Agency

The development of agentic processes in Angelique's life-history originates upon the foundation of the Maternal Ground. The agentic postures of Angelique's developing ego and self, which stem from the dwelling and inhabiting enactments of the Maternal, create the possibility for Angelique's action. Angelique's agency is directed toward her life goals, and it manifests itself frequently as life-affirming expressions—expressions of her emotional states, self-efficacy, independence, authority, and identity—or, in later moments, as palliative responses to her pain and suffering. The temporal dimensions of agency involve past retentions, the present state, and the futural horizon of experience.

Angelique's inexorable drive moves her toward her intended and determinate goals and a fulfilling agency to help satisfy her intentions and meanings. In Angelique engages in agentic processes that reveal a relationship between the Maternal Ground and her own experience of suffering. Her practical agentic processes involve the use of equipment, such as eating, toileting, therapy, and taking medications. Other equally meaningful agentic processes in which she is involved, although less visible, are communication with staff in the care facility in her activities of daily living, seeking empathic care in relationships with family members and health professionals, her spiritual reflections and engagements, situating herself in a secure and comfortable dwelling place, and finding resolution in a final place of rest. Some of these agentic processes involve projective capacities and intentions with futural horizons, and the use of imagination to enable Angelique to configure a vision of what the future will hold for her. She describes a future in a place like her native islands, where she will enjoy sociality, relationality, and relief from suffering.

The field of practical action involving use of equipment demonstrates Angelique's effective agency, such as in the area of eating. Even though Angelique cannot feed herself and requires assistance, her self-agency is not reducible to bodily movement. For example, she has a desire for tea, and she will request it from the staff if she is not served a cup:

> No, I am not really hungry because I drink a cup of tea. Yes, I love tea. Breakfast they give me a cup; lunch they give me a cup. Supper they give me a cup. … I have to ask for a cup if they don't remember to put it on my tray. I remind them.

This fulfilling experience enhances Angelique's perceptions of self-efficacy, an embodiment of the Maternal dimensions of existence and an expression of meaning, emotion, and value. She enjoys it. Angelique's agency, when actualized, results in feeling at home in a situation that fulfills her desires.

Angelique employs a different type of agentic process when it comes to eating at the care facility: a process of resistance. Her general unhappiness with the lived experience of eating is directed toward her quality of life. Her active resistance to the care facility's delivery of care in this area, expressed through expressive and non-expressive communication, is an example of her powerful sense of agency:

> Now today they had macaroni with beef, something thrown over it. So when I got to the table, that's what was there. … I said I didn't want it. … "What you want?" they say. I say, "You know I eat chicken." And I am sure they have chicken, but every day they say one more [day]. So I didn't take it. So the guy came to pick it up. … When I went back to the table, they say "She give you chicken." But what kind of chicken? A piece of chicken? Hard.
>
> So I left it right there. I didn't eat nothing. So I didn't eat lunch. But I am not hungry because I drank that cup of tea. I had the tea. Yes, right and I find the tea very soothing.
>
> … My meals have been paid for before I walk in this place, which is correct. … They pay for my meal before anything else. So we should get sometime, you see, breakfast once, one slice of toast, cup of tea.
>
> There were no eggs. I like our eggs. Not what they call their eggs. … Let me make it myself. … Yes, I was a cook. Eating's not bad. Every day the meals get less and less. They give little food. I am hungry. No, I don't find the food comforting.

Angelique does not want the hard piece of chicken, and she refuses it. She experiences the chicken as non-Maternal, in stark contrast to the soothing tea. She understands and enacts the agency of refusal. This self-agency has important implications for refusing treatment options, as the process of choosing, deliberation, and making judgments about health care treatment may share some of the same cognitive and affective characteristics.

The strong sense of agency that Angelique describes over her bodily movements is distinct from ownership of the bodily movement itself. She shares a moment during which one of her daughters bathes her, and she describes being able to stand to allow herself to be properly washed. Angelique sustains a desire for mobility and communicates a sense of achievement at being able to complete the task of standing in an upright position for the purpose of the washing:

> Yes, they have to help me. I am able to stand when she washes me. Yes, but my daughter herself doesn't like it. She doesn't like to wash me up. The other granddaughter could do it in a wink. But this is L, the one who could do it.

Crucially, the Maternal contains a duality of lived experience in which agentic and non-agentic processes coexist. Non-agentic processes co-occur with the agentic. Angelique exists in the Maternal, where she receives compassionate loving care. While she makes an agentic decision to be in relation with her caregiver to receive this care, she also removes herself from agentic processes in the manner of how she passively receives the care itself. This move from active to passive agency is a critical developmental milestone at the end of life, as it prepares the seriously ill person for the ultimate passivity and letting go, which is death. In Angelique's dependency on others for comfort, she is not without agency, and she forms a cooperative, collaborative relationship with the caregiver that is crucial to the reestablishment of the Maternal Ground.

Social contexts of agency and social systems

Angelique effuses glowingly about accomplishing the task of holding her granddaughter's newborn baby, a task that is socially and relationally situated. The achievement of being a great-grandmother, taking the baby in her arms, and sharing this joy with her family members displays the great emotional value and significance Angelique attaches to these experiences and to her self-agency. Her sense of self-agency here goes beyond bodily movement and extends to the Maternal dimensions of her role in the family, her continuing achievement of the tasks associated with the Maternal role, and her bringing to bear tasks already accomplished throughout her life history.

Angelique shows evidence of the futural horizons of agency, as well as other complex aspects of agency. She draws upon her projective capacities to imagine and configure a place of rest and rescue to which she can retreat as she approaches the end of her life:

I'm here. And right now, I'm thinking of something that I want. I want to leave here. No. Get a different place. Mm-hmm. I'm hoping. And praying. Yeah, and that's what I am asking God for. That I'll have somebody there…

You know, a woman. No man. I'm done with them. A companion. Just that when you come in, you could say, "Hi. How have you been today?" And she'll answer you, and you'll answer her back. Go eat dinner together. … So I'm looking forward. Mm-hmm. I can't even talk with my daughter, she's so busy working.

No. So I'll see what the Master can do for me. … One of these days, He will grant my wish. Yes. When He sees right.

… No longer than this week, I said to the oldest daughter, "I thank you for not having enough time to even see me."

I come in at night at 6:30. She [care facility staff] tell them, "Give her a shower and put her to bed." I don't feel like I want to go to bed at 6:30; 6:30 is kind of early. I have to go to bed at 6:30. Right, no choice. Mm-hmm. … My family didn't trust me living by myself anymore. They took the keys. They took the lock, everything. … What I want, I really want to come up, take my shoes off, throw myself across the bed and relax. I don't go places. Nothing. And that's how I feel. They keep saying, "Mammy, this is good for you." It's good for them. It's not good for me. … It might be good for them as they feel that I would have company, but it's not for me. It's not good for me. I like to know I could come here, or wherever I am, I could come up, put on some clothes or take off my clothes. Sit up until I … see, me going to bed at 6:30 at nighttime, I don't like it.

The intentionality of action present in Angelique's future orientation is necessary to the agentic process. She holds a dream with a focus on striving to achieve the possibilities of the future—reminiscent of Dr. Martin Luther King Jr.'s famous dream in its themes of free agency, freedom, and liberation. Full of intention, Angelique wills the possible and directs her agency toward a sure and determinate goal. She seeks a Maternal homecoming, along with the potentialities that constitute the Maternal system in a futural horizon: relational intimacy and care, autonomy, and existential and spiritual transcendence. Although the goal is certain and determinate, the route to achieving it is not, and Angelique's self-agency and circumstances may not be sufficient to fulfilling it.

Angelique's wishes and her disappointments reveal a number of other aspects of agency at work. She takes practical action in her current situation and in the iterational aspects of narrative. At least four levels of action can be disaggregated within the unity of temporality in this description. Angelique's prayerful activity in the present moment is directed toward the goal of moving to a different place and finding companionship—a goal achieved through prayerful action. Angelique also makes an appeal to her daughter to rescue her, staking a moral claim. She engages in tactics of resistance—rejecting the order the care facility imposes upon her with respect to such everyday activities as what time to go to bed and when to take off her clothes. Again, here too co-occurrent agentic and non-agentic processes manifest in Angelique's actions, which means that certain aspects of Angelique's social processes, such as the rescue itself, do not involve self-agency.

The care Angelique describes has two constituents: goodness and moral responsibility. The Maternal care she has provided to her family in the past is essentially good, having as its only goal the producing of good. Angelique takes up moral agency in passive syntheses and recollections, as well as through re-enactments, informed by her history of belonging to a family and a community in her early and adult life. The Maternal and ethical dimensions of family and community retained in Angelique's horizon structure, combined with her resilience in the face of the hardships sustained throughout her life and the stalwart, independent disposition she developed through these experiences, have made Angelique a strong moral agent. She makes a moral commitment to her relational others in her Maternal, caring, dispositional, and agentic roles. Angelique spends a great deal of time describing her Maternal role and the hard work it entails through practices such as sewing, cooking, making birthday cakes, and taking good care of her children and meaningful others under great financial hardship as a widow and single mother.

Angelique desires to return at the end of her life to her origin, Maternal roots, and home:

> Of course I do have a desire to return to the islands. I've been back several times. The islands. I was born there. I was there when the volcano came. … I just feel—I tell her, sometime maybe when you come, you won't even find me. Yeah. That's right. Imagine that I'm in the islands. … I think about when I was growing up there. Yes, it was lovely. You had to work hard. It wasn't then no big money, but you had to work. And that's what you had to do to eat.
>
> Think of images of the islands, how you can come outside and sit down, and nobody bother you. … Thinking about a special place that I would like to go to. Yeah, the islands. My daughters are saying no, but they don't want me to leave them, too. Yes, I've told them I would like to go back to the islands. … "Mammy, you're in the best place." I say, "Yes, the best place when you think so. When I don't think so. I know it's not the best place for me." That's where I was born, in the islands. And that's where I lived until I left the home there.

Angelique's reflections and imaginative variations reveal an agentic, projective process directed toward seeking a place of rest in the setting of Maternal origin. Angelique not only seeks rescue and relief from her suffering, but actively engages in that process through an imaginative configuration of her place of rest. In her ethical relation with her daughters, she makes a moral claim on them as agents, who have a moral responsibility to her to help provide the rescue she needs.

Spirituality

For Angelique, the Maternal Ground provides the foundation for her spirituality. Religion, as a formal structure, has formal belief systems as its foundation. Religion and spirituality overlap in Angelique's testimony, but they are distinct systems. There is a duality of lived experience for Angelique in her experience of spirituality, which is itself rooted in the Maternal dimensions of existence. Spirituality overlaps with suffering: it arises even in the presence of suffering. Is it possible for Angelique to experience suffering in the total absence of spirituality? The Maternal Ground, and spirituality that is founded on the Maternal Ground, are conditions for the possibility of suffering, just as they are conditions for the possibility of development and fulfillment. Without the presence of spirituality, there is no possibility for losses of the Maternal Foundations that are an invariant of the structure of suffering. Angelique is spiritual and has a consciousness of her spirituality. She also has a consciousness of suffering, and she holds her spiritual and suffering experiences at the same time.

The Maternal Ground also founds agency. Parallel to experiences of suffering, the systems of spirituality and agency overlap, but Angelique's spirituality does not collapse in the face of co-occurrent agentic and non-agentic processes at work. She demonstrates agency in response to her suffering while also living through her suffering and experiencing disabled agency in certain domains of her life.

Angelique's spirituality can act to expand, strengthen, and enable agency. Conversely, desire and agency can strengthen spirituality. Angelique, as a moral agent, seeks good food, good friendship, good health care, good toileting, and good communication in the care facility, but also seeks fulfillment of higher-order spiritual needs. Angelique desires to think about things in the "right" way—to make the right choices and decisions in her practical moral life, and to have appropriate responses in her situation in the care facility and in her vocational projects in the world, such as her projects of providing Maternal care and nourishment. In this way, Angelique seeks the essential spiritual goods of an inter-subjectively experienced agency. Her agency expands her intentional spiritual movement toward the good.

How do these systems and the complex of relationships among these systems manifest themselves in Angelique's life? Angelique's testimony provides evidence of her very powerful spiritual intentionalities in both visible and non-visible ways. For Angelique, spirituality discloses itself as a connectedness to things outside and beyond the self—to God, to the Maternal, to her origin, and to other people. This sustaining source of strength is temporally embedded in lived experience, yet transcends experience and existence. The experience of spirituality opens up the possibility for Angelique to recover the agency partially disabled by her illness, pain, and suffering. Her spiritual intentionalities remove barriers to the fulfillment of the meaning of her intentions, and they help her to locate her place in time and space and to find rest. The spiritual affirms Angelique's dignity and restores her to existential wholeness. The experience of the spiritual has strong affective dimensions. Angelique's emotional responses of hope and joy in the experience of spirituality disclose the values that are meaningful to her in her end-of-life decision making: fidelity, trust, and empathic care.

The systems of religion and spirituality have nuanced and subtle differentiations of meaning, although the two have fluid boundaries. One distinction concerns the spiritual care provided to Angelique by the professional staff of the care facility through formal systems and structures; another concerns spirituality and spiritual meanings arising in relationships with relational others including family members; a third domain is the spirituality embedded in Angelique's life history and social and cultural contexts; and a fourth is Angelique's own personal spiritual movement and flourishing. There is variation, spatially and temporally, in the pervasiveness of spirituality and religion in each of these respective domains. Generally, spirituality is the more pervasive experience for Angelique.

Angelique describes the spiritual needs that arise from her existential situation in the care facility, depending on her family for care, and not having her spiritual needs adequately addressed by the professional staff in the care facility. She feels that the staff responsible for her spiritual care have not formed interpersonal relationships with her that have meaning in her quest for spiritual nourishment, independent of whether she has been provided with services by such staff. She does not receive the care from the staff that she seeks in order to satisfy her deeply spiritual personal inclinations, her desires for connectivity to something outside herself, and her need to understand and motivate a recovery from suffering and helplessness:

> Nobody talks to me about my spiritual needs. A lady, she's an Adventist and she works there. And one day I met her and I say "Howdy-do" to her and she say, "Howdy-do," and she say, "Where do you live?" I showed her where I live, you know, told her. She say, "Okay, I'm going to come see you"—but she never showed up. She never showed up, so. … You have to make life the best way you could, right? I think that some of the people have it harder than I do, but I still think mine is hard enough.
>
> And with my children and grandchildren, it's not much help, because they have to take care of their children. And I don't—I didn't ask that I would be resting on them like this. But this is life and we have to face it.

Angelique's personal desires, inclinations, and goal-directed behaviors to create connectedness are well established her rootedness in the volcanic soil, hurricane waters, and river of the islands, in the home she built to raise her children, in her ties to family—her mother, grandmother, and great-grandmother, her brother, her aunt, and her daughters and their progeny —and through her faith in God.

Finally, Angelique expresses a desire to have rest from her suffering. Her desire and enactments have a teleological aspect that is deeply spiritual in nature. She speaks of putting in a good day, of always doing her best to serve her children, of having it "hard enough," of relieving the burden she places on her relational others, of making sure everything is in order before she dies, and of returning to a place where she will find the rest she seeks. She prays and hopes for a place where she can share even the simplest, most everyday things with a companion. She expresses a desire for sociality in this place of rest. The special place she envisions going to is her native islands, where she can go outside and have people greet her. These descriptions of her final resting place share the character of being intersubjectively experienced, interembodied, other-regarding, and Maternally cradling. Angelique's end of life remains full of possibility—open to new lived experiences and growth. Angelique's testimony makes transparent that suffering and spirituality share space in her life-world. As she moves toward the end of life and dwells more on her desire and enactments toward returning home and finding rest, her spirituality expands spatially and temporally to help her achieve the developmental milestones that bring relief to her suffering condition.

Religion

Angelique is spiritually centered, and she also has a very powerful faith in the God of her religion. She observes her religion, a formal system of beliefs, through membership in a church community and in cultural tradition and practice. Religion and spirituality do not conflict, nor do they conflict with her agency—although there is the potential for such conflict. Her religion and spirituality both act to enable her development and resilience in the alienating environment of the care facility. Each also enables her recovery of the Maternal dimensions of existence and agency, creating the possibility for transcendence. Reciprocally, Angelique's desire and agency propel intentional spiritual movement.

In her everyday speech, Angelique expresses a strong faith in and fidelity to God, and a belief that God watches over her and will call her home. Her faith sustains her:

> I love when my family comes to see me. Makes you feel good. Anyway, one of these days the Good Lord is going to call and take me home. And I won't be here to bother with them. But they're all right. They're not too bad. My first daughter is up there over there [looking at picture on wall].
>
> And then they [family members] start coming and they are not able to stop in. Anyway, God knows what he's doing.
>
> I worry about them [family members] in a way… I can't tell where they are, what they're doing. I don't want to be a burden to her [daughter]. Because, you know, her daughter is twenty years and she [is] making a baby. But God will watch over us.

This strong faith in God, embedded in Angelique's early childhood experiences growing up in the islands with her mother, spans her lifetime. Her faith is life-historical—deeply rooted in community and in her religion. Her mother took her to church when she was a child and taught her to pray. She belonged to a church community. Angelique followed these same religious practices with her own children as members of a community. She believes that if she prays to God, her wishes will be granted. Her religion is a formal structure in her lived experience that serves as a source of sustained strength for her in the face of enduring hardship and suffering. Angelique oftentimes turns to her religion when no other personal or interpersonal resources are available to her, and when she has limited access to the type of relational care that she seeks with family members and non-family caregivers. In the depths of her moral displacement and sense of homelessness, Angelique turns to her faith in God as a delivery from suffering.

The meaning of this faith in God, however, surpasses the meaning of religion for Angelique. Her experience of faith and of God personally has mystical dimensions. She experiences this faith intuitively, as a given, and in that givenness she experiences a union with God. She describes this union as a self-initiated experience:

Anyway, God is good. He'll watch over you if you put yourself in the way.

Angelique suggests an active process, a self-agency in which she exposes herself to God. This experience has both active and passive dimensions—active agency in exposing herself to God, but passive in allowing God to become present in her life. This form of agency—which does not require any worldly power, physical effectiveness, or social support—in particular helps Angelique in facing suffering when other forms of agency fail.

The "chicken head" episode is illustrative of the type of experience Angelique had in the central temporal moment of her life history when she had lost her Maternal Foundations and had difficulty in transitioning to an attitude of praxis toward the world. The constituents of suffering in the individual structure that arose in this temporal moment were losses of dignity, self, humanity, role, autonomy, self-efficacy, and fulfilling agency; losses of the welcoming home, boundaries, and family and social structures; losses of sociality and community, relational discontinuity with family members, and the absence of meaningful relationships with professional caregivers; accumulation of burden, and a pervasive sense of affliction in her end-of-life illness from which there was no relief or rescue.

In the midst of and alongside this suffering, Angelique also exhibits a desire to detach herself from suffering, beginning with an agentic stance. She proclaims a desire to walk after going on hospice, defying her state of affairs as a person with a terminal diagnosis who was no longer receiving restorative care. She projects her futural horizon in a place in which she would be free of pain and enjoys sociality. She is sustained by her spirituality and her religion, and by a powerful desire to be agentic that was also rooted in the Maternal Ground. The origin of the horizon of experience is rooted in the Maternal system and relation. Angelique's experience of the Maternal dimensions of existence temporally preceded her experiences of suffering and her fall from height—from the security and comfort of the Maternal. In this way, consciousness of suffering expanded her consciousness of the possibility of something other than suffering, namely, the good, pursuit of the good as a moral agent, and the achievement of some modicum of well-being.

Angelique does not collapse under her suffering. Suffering and spirituality co-exist in Angelique's life-world. Angelique's harkening back to the place where she was born expands her deeply spiritual lived experiences of receiving care and being rooted in a home, and disclose her teleological desire for and movement toward a Maternal homecoming and resting place at the end of life. This resting place is relationally constituted. Angelique imagines the fulfillment of her desires for meaning in a futural horizon where she would be free of pain and return to the enjoyment of the world as she recalled it from her early life in the islands. There is an existential transcendence and resurrection in this teleological movement, and a joyful and celebratory character to her resting place. Angelique is reflective and thankful for the good life she has led and for all her blessings. She anticipates achieving fulfillment of meanings in a future that would be made possible by her agency and the movement of her spiritual intentionalities toward a Maternal homecoming.

Conclusion

In the third temporal moment of suffering, Angelique experiences a self-actualizing movement toward a recovery of agency and well-being, and a journeying toward a Maternal homecoming at the end of life. Her decision making manifests itself as a resilient social and spiritual process and expression of agency in response to her suffering, through which she draws upon multiple resources. The flow of temporal moments and the developmental structure of suffering and decision making have plasticity, and permit Angelique to accommodate change in her environment. Empathic care and spiritual well-being are important eidetic meanings in Angelique's life-world as she struggles to live with life-threatening illness and imagines a hopeful future in a final place of rest. Angelique's spiritual movement in this third temporal moment is consistent with what John Drummond (2008a) describes in moral phenomenology as the shift from the pursuit of the visible or manifest material goods of agency, to the higher-order, non-manifest spiritual goods of agency itself.

Suffering among seriously ill elderly persons is a multidimensional personal and intersubjective experience that implicates a person's social ecology, web of social relationships, and developmental history. The Maternal Ground, along with its manifestations of agency and instantiations in person decision making and other variegated forms, can act as palliative responses to suffering that permit seriously ill persons to recover lost Maternal Foundations and re-establish the constitutive empathy, comfort, and security of the Maternal Ground. Phenomenological analysis supports that goodness is invariant in the Maternal— which is not inconsistent with empirical examples of acts of "mothering" that may demonstrate the privative of the Maternal.

5 The Narrative of Camila

Enacting and Re-Enacting Cultural Meanings of Faith and Fidelity

Cultural meanings of faith and fidelity figured prominently in the life history of "Camila," an 86-year-old Latina widow admitted to the care facility over a decade ago. Camila resided in the long-term care unit and was eventually moved into a single room. She had no children, but she did have very involved family members. She had both a Do Not Resuscitate Order and a health care surrogate. Although she had multiple chronic illnesses including diagnoses of hypertension, chronic kidney disease, angina, peripheral vascular disease, and other co-morbid conditions, Camila was independent in her activities of daily living, and enjoyed participating in group recreation such as bingo. She ambulated with a walker, but was remarkably mobile in navigating the long halls of the care facility. I conducted six interviews with Camila.

During one of my visits to see her, Camila seemed very unsettled. She told me that she was involved in an unpleasant encounter with another resident. This encounter assumed prominence in Camila's experience of suffering. Not long after, Camila told me she had been transferred to a hospital for a psychiatric evaluation because of the same incident with her fellow resident. The medical record documented that Camila hit another resident in the face because the resident was saying things about Camila's mother that Camila felt were not only unacceptable, but also an assault on the most sacred cultural meanings of the iconic mother figure that she held dear. Camila was transferred back to the care facility by ambulette the same day.

Synthesis and Founding Order of Camila's Individual Structure of Suffering

Like "Angelique," Camila experienced suffering in an individual structure constituted by three temporal moments. In a first temporal moment, the Maternal Ground and its constituents found other prominent features of lived experience in suffering—including agency, sociality, and spirituality. In a second temporal moment, Camila is thrown into a vortex of pain and suffering. Finally, she moves toward a recovery of agency. Camila's relational decision making is also founded upon the Maternal, and communication is in turn founded upon relationality.

Cultural meanings, cultural forms of communication, and culturally sensitive care responses to the seriously ill elderly person are salient in this individual structure.

First Temporal Moment: Maternal Ground and Origin of Horizon of Experience

Camila's lived experiences are deeply rooted in Maternal dimensions of existence and her early life experiences in her native country with her mother, home, and in a family of cultural origin. It is in the Maternal realm that she develops a sense of inhabiting the world, a stance of active agency toward the world, and a love for life that are motivated by a desire for otherness, and self-actualization. The Maternal Ground and its essential constituents lay a foundation for the development of full relationality with others in the world. In her relationships with her family and her husband, and in her work, Camila is relation-centered:

> Sometimes I think about my mother and my father and my husband, which are my darlings, but they are gone. They are gone. It's nothing we can do. It's in the hands of God whatever happens, yeah.

Camila brings her past retentions of profound love from her mother, and faithful care in a welcoming home environment, to bear in her current horizons. These retentions shape her life and her attitude toward the world, others in the world, and her drive to achieve an overall sense of well-being—even when challenged by her current environment in the care facility. Camila reflects on both her mother's grieving upon her departure from the family home and her mother's death soon thereafter:

> My mother almost cried, and she says, "I will die without my child. I will die without her." My mother, she died. She had a heart attack, yes. And she died because she said she couldn't bear to have myself being the oldest of the children being out of the house. During that time if you were single, you did not live out of their mother and their father house, it was different.

The loss of her mother is a traumatic event in Camila's life that has multidimensional meanings for her. She suggests a causal relationship between her departure from the ancestral home and her mother's death. She feels she is the reason for her mother's death, and she feels responsible for her mother's death. But the loss of her mother takes on a significance that founds other meanings and experiences in her life. It becomes a thematic structure in her experience that is temporally embedded in her intentionalities.

Seeking Well-Being in the Home as Dwelling, Inhabiting, Welcoming Hospitality, Protective Environment, Nourishment, and Origin

Camila's move from her own home and dwelling to the care facility precipitates a number of shifts in attitude about the home. At first, when she transitions to the care facility, she is disoriented, dislocated, and feeling displaced and unwelcome in a foreign environment—especially after the devastating loss of her husband and having to give up her own apartment and home:

> I felt very horrible [about giving up my apartment]. I thought I died. I thought I died. Living in that apartment for twenty-four years that was like my own home, but naturally I was paying my rent there. But this was happen, that my family said that I could not take care of it anymore; I couldn't do the cleaning anymore because I was 77 years old. "Why don't you rest?" they say. "You have worked enough."
>
> I worked for 40 years. Forty years. "You have worked enough. You don't need the money. We will give you everything you need, plus you have your own security. Your insurance has done everything. You don't need no money, nothing. You need money, there is a bank downstairs that you can withdraw money. There will always be money in there for you and that's it."
>
> In the beginning, making the transition was terrible. I didn't want to eat. I didn't want to talk to nobody. I didn't want to talk to nobody. I didn't want to see my family. I didn't want to go to the dining room. I didn't want to do—to do nothing, just staring up in the bed, staring up, staring up, staring up.

However, over time Camila expands her shrunken spatiality and temporality and carves out a new place of dwelling in the care facility. She has a desire to go places and widen her field of vision and experience. While some people and parts of the world still remain foreign and alien to her, she is continually renegotiating the boundaries of space, pushing outward and inhabiting new worlds. The non-home, non-dwelling or realm outside the home that is foreign and alienating always remains in view and open to exploration. In the spirit of Woolf (1957), Camila establishes a "room of her own" within the care facility that is her private dwelling and in which she conducts her everyday routines of bathing, toileting, dressing, and daily praying the rosary in Spanish. These are agentic activities of a habitual nature that are not reflective. In her room, she seeks the comfort, security, hospitality, and well-being of the Maternal relation that she recalls from her past experiences. Beyond a room that she has made her own, she makes regular and daily forays into the world—going places both within the care facility through activities, meals, and interactions with residents and health care professionals, and going on excursions outside the four walls of the home to the baseball stadium and the botanical garden, and reading the newspapers to discover more about her neighbors in the world and their life situations. She reveals a healthy openness to others and a thirst for new experiences, a desire to expand the boundaries of her life-world.

Seeking Independence and Care Through Desire and Agency

The constituents of desire and agency are central to understanding Camila's lived experiences at the end of life. Both desire and agency are social and relational and are intentional movements that are emotional in character. These constituents have their origin in the Maternal experience and the dwelling and relational intimacy with the mother. The desire for otherness, union with the other, and exteriority begins in the Maternal experience. Camila seeks the security and comfort of the Maternal holding environment in her relationship with her psychologist. Camila has a very strong desire for independence and for health and well-being:

> I am independent. I am independent. It is very important to me. Independence. Independence. Independent. I do my own—my own cleaning. I do my own—I dress myself. I feed myself. I know what I want. I read the news every morning, 7:00. At 7:00 sharp I come down from my floor. I come here to the security desk and say, "Will you please give me my paper?" I pay $9.99 for that paper a month. Yes. I have to read. Otherwise I be dead. Why is that—I mean, what's the sense of living if you don't take part of what's going on in your country? I have to feel care—connected, that I know what's going on. I know. How can I live like a parasite? I don't want to live like a parasite. First I want to live like a person. I have to know what's going on. When is night and when is day?
>
> That's the way I feel. I don't know.

Agency is a temporally embedded enactment, performance, or achievement that is directed toward a goal. Camila takes up her desire for independence in agentic processes through intentional action. She does things—dresses herself, feeds herself, does her own cleaning. She goes to the security desk to get her newspaper. She reads the news. She goes about her business in light of the aims she has to be connected and to "feel care." Camila seeks a fulfilling agency that will satisfy the meanings of her intentions to be in social engagement with the world.

Relational Intimacy

Camila's relation-centered attitude is revealed in the narrative data in her recall of past experiences of relationships with her mother, her father, her husband, and her experiences of their dying; in her relationships with her siblings and their children, with her nurse practitioner and psychologist; and with at least two of the residents in the care facility. She seeks intimate sharing with others in her relationships. These relationships involve sharing experiences over a span of time. Relationality also has a strong ethical dimension for her. The ethical relation is constitutive of the Maternal. The ground of obligation for moral action as Camila perceives it is moral responsibility to the other. Camila perceives that her professional caregivers stand in ethical relation to her, and she draws upon her past experiences of the ethical and moral responsibility in relationships with family to make moral claims upon her caregivers for empathic care.

Camila communicates her lived-through experiences of being profoundly loved—first by a loving, faithful, and caring mother, then by a father who was devoted to her mother, and finally by a husband who was also steadfast in his devotion even in his last months of life. Camila's mother died a premature death in her early fifties, and therefore cut short Camila's life experience with her in early adulthood. Camila experiences her mother's death as a kind of death herself. But she appropriates her mother's dying and makes the Maternal a foundation of her lived experiences and, more importantly, her agency. She takes on a Maternal role in the family as the head of the household and the expanded family, and provides nurturing, loving care to her father, her siblings and their children, and her spouse. Camila understands the constituents of the Maternal as dwelling, intimate relational sharing, fidelity, and compassionate, loving care, and she makes the pursuit of these virtues and qualities central to her life. These agentic processes motivate and drive the care she provides to her father at the end of his life, taking the place of her mother and creating a homelike, welcoming environment for him in the family when he is transplanted from his native islands to the States—a place that he finds cold and unwelcoming. These agentic processes also found her expectations for empathic care in her current situation in the care facility. Camila's relationship with her husband stands out as existentially, spiritually, and temporally transcendent. She is deeply and spiritually connected with him in life and in death, as well as in life after death:

> When I was—it was on account of the death of my husband. I mean, don't forget, we were married many years, and that is not easy to forget. Still, I think of him. I still sometimes go to sleep and I see him.
>
> Yes, I dream a lot about him. We were together for so many years. And we grew up together. We went to school together. That was my childhood sweetheart. So you can imagine I cannot forget him. Since that, I never looked on other men. Nobody is equal to him, to me. Now, I'm always finding faults. I don't know. That's the way it is. Other people, right away they say, "Okay, I will look for somebody else right away so I can forget." No, I don't. I don't want to forget. He was good to me, so why should I share him with somebody? No. That's not for me.
>
> Otherwise, I feel all right. And after that, everybody, the psychologist, they came to visit me and everything. They thought, you know—preach at me, "Camila, you have to eat. Camila, you have to meet people. You have to talk to people. You have to forget your past. The past is gone. Be on your senses."

This connectedness is a phenomenon that is beyond the existential relational self and signifies a "surplus" in the nature of the infinite. In her thoughts, Camila's husband constantly is present to her. She sees him coming to her in her dreams and sees herself always being in his embrace. She is always faithful to him. This fidelity is rooted in the Maternal. Camila recalls her past experiences of Maternal care and how she incorporated them into her agentic caring process toward her husband. When her husband was dying and experiencing excruciating pain from cancer, she soothed him and helped him understand why it was acceptable for him to take pain medications to relieve his pain, and she experienced a reciprocal devotion from him even as he lay dying. He survived his end-of-life illness for a year and a half and put things in order for her before he died.

Camila's relational commitments extend to her siblings and their children. She assumes responsibility for them after her mother's death, consistent with what she saw as the cultural expectations of the Maternal role and Maternal duties. She is the head of the household and the "second mother" for her brothers, nieces, and nephews. Serving in this role does not detract from the relational meaning in the interpersonal relationships she has with each loved member of her family.

In the care facility setting, Camila develops meaningful relationships with two health care professionals in particular: her nurse practitioner (whom she refers to as her doctor) and her psychologist. She expresses confidence in each of these members of the interdisciplinary team and the good care they provide to her. She also expresses a generally positive attitude toward her social worker, but does not express a need for her services and does not seem to have a relational intimacy with her. Camila seems to have the closest relational intimacy with her psychologist, whom she describes as "like a mother," and with whom she is comfortable sharing things. Given Camila's reverence for the Maternal, this description of her psychologist and what she means to her is significant. Camila's ability to reverse roles and receive the Maternal in a meaningful interpersonal relationship provides evidence of her enormous capacity for growth, recovery of agency, and resilience.

Although Camila experiences certain barriers to forming friendships and relationships with other residents in the care facility, she does describe meaningful relationships with her friend, J, who has passed away, and her Cuban friend, M. Relationships with other residents in the care facility are important to Camila and she values these relationships. She suffers deeply from the loss of her friend J. She relishes the companionship of her friend M. When she has an unexpected incident with a resident who calls her an unacceptable name that suggests irreverence for her mother, she is deeply hurt and offended. She cannot make meaning of such irreverence within her cultural experience and has a violent reaction to it. The absence of deep relational connections with other residents in the care facility is a source of suffering for Camila. She feels the absence of these connections because she is relation-centered. Cultural barriers—such as the lack of commonalities in language, tastes in food, and habits and practices—heighten Camila's feeling of being separated from others in the care facility.

Communication

Camila reveals that she is motivated by a desire for interpersonal conversation and communication. She communicates through language and other forms of expressive communication in intimate relations. Her communication is founded upon the interpersonal relationships she establishes with others—family members, her spouse, health care professionals, and other residents. There is also evidence of mutuality and reciprocity in her relational communication with others— although this is not a necessary or sufficient condition of such relationships.

Culture

The Maternal Ground also founds culture. The relationship of culture to the other constituents in the individual structure involves complexity. Culture can run afferently from the external macro system to the personal system, or efferently from the personal system to the external system. The defining of culture in this research investigation is from Camila's first-person personal system perspective— an insider's perspective. Throughout the narrative data, Camila makes the issues of her cultural origin and her cultural experience thematic. She first describes the mother as an iconic figure in her culture and the reverence and sacred treatment of the mother. The meanings of the Maternal for her are love, fidelity, relation-centeredness, and care. Camila gives primacy to the mother in her structure of the family and her structure of the world. She also describes the family in her Latina culture and what family means in her culture, especially in the context of providing care. The family also has primacy in Camila's culture. She gives testimony about how her husband understood that her family and the needs of her family had priority over his needs. Her decision not to have a child also provides evidence of the importance of the family of cultural origin for her. Camila's account of the care she and her siblings provided to her father when he was dying provides further evidence of cultural expectations of the family's commitment to taking care of elders.

In these accounts, Camila conveys a strong sense of cultural identity. She was born outside the borders of the United States, but she expresses an abiding love for America and describes America in Maternal terms. She seeks out the company of other residents in the care facility who share cultural commonalities with her such as common language, common tastes in food, common manners; forms of respect for others; and values, prayers, and icons, although she takes pleasure in associating with the Italians and the Irish as well. She experiences disappointment and a sense of shrunken spatiality when she does not have the opportunity to form friendships with other residents who share such commonalities, habits, and practices:

> So, I stayed here, and here I am, nine years, and everything is all right except—I mean, when you live in a place where you have to get along with these people that are not from—first of all, they're not from your own race, and secondly, they don't have your own—your own schooling. They don't have anything in common with you, and I don't have nothing in common with them. You have to adapt—trying to adapt little by little with these people, as long as they have to be adapted to myself also, to know me. And that's it. Everything is all right. I been here nine years. My family comes to visit me every other week, and I have everything. I live all right.

To this extent, culture is a barrier for her in her home space and limits her expansion into the zone outside the home. Camila's experience of the absence of understanding of cultural differences by the staff of the care facility, or any attempt on their part to negotiate cultural differences and conflicts, stands as both a relational and a communication barrier to her well-being and comfort in the care facility and her relational decision making.

Spirituality

Camila has an abiding faith in God that she feels is empowering, and a source of strength and enjoyment for her. God provides a good life and helps her to actualize her sense of agency. This faith is also a ground of obligation for moral action:

> I have my faith that is before anything. That sustains me. . . I am very proud of my age. Thanks to God. Before anything, I thank God that he's the one that keeps me alive. I feel everything—if I didn't have no faith I think I'd rather be dead. I need my faith. I go to mass. I take my sacred communion every week, and I feel wonderful. I thank God every day and every night for everything I have. I have so much. Others don't have nothing, and I have so much. I thank God. I thank God I have too much. Yes.

Beyond this faith, which is governed by a formal system of beliefs to which Camila assents, she is also spiritually-centered—that is, connected with something beyond herself that is central in her life and a source of sustaining strength in the face of challenges—God is with her and present in her life and who discloses the beauty in the world. Spirituality takes in Camila's connectedness to relational others whose experiences she inhabits or with whom she has relational intimacy, and it shapes her life-world both spatially and temporally. Her connectedness with her husband is such an example. Even after his death, she carries him with her in her thoughts and her living in the world. He is always present to her. Camila's connectedness to her origin—the Maternal—also has a spiritual character. Spirituality is a broader concept than faith and is not a formal system of beliefs. Camila's embracing of faith and spirituality is contingent upon agency and a desire for self-actualization, but can also help to strengthen and recover a sense of agency and help to actualize it. Desire and agency themselves are essential constituents of the Maternal structure. As founding of culture and spirituality, the Maternal Ground and its constituents of home and desire and agency are also essential aspects of spirituality. There is a relationship between spirituality and the agentic stance of inhabiting and dwelling, and of openness to possibility, growth, and self-actualization. Camila prays in her native language and the prayers have a cultural meaning for her:

> I have rosary beads in my room. I use them every day. Yes, every day. No, no, not special. Just Catholic. Catholic rosary. Yeah. I say most of it, half of it, I do it. I do the rosary complete. Completely. I'm used to. I'm used to, yes.

Santa Maria is mother in Spanish. Everything in Spanish. It is amazing. But I need it. If I don't do it, I feel like I am incomplete. Like I am missing something, that God is going to punish me, anyway. I said, "No, no, no, no, no, I can't go without it." I have to do it. I have to do it. Every morning. Yes, it's part of my routine. And at night, when I go to sleep, I do part of it.

Camila has clear spiritual intentionalities that are directed toward her relationship with God, and she prays to fulfill the meaning of her intentionalities. Her prayerful action is a powerful form of self-agency. Spirituality is a multidimensional experience, and has strong affective dimensions. Camila demonstrates emotional responses to her faith and spiritual experiences that disclose the values she attaches to her experiences and conflicts in values.

Spirituality and agency came into conflict for Camila when she made a decision not to have a child, even after becoming pregnant. Her faith and the beliefs of her faith dictated that she ought to keep her baby. However, she had a strong sense of agency—practical agency—and emotional responses to practical concerns that disclosed values that attached more significance to work, economic security and independence, and taking care of her extended family. She did not have the financial resources that would permit supporting a child of her own. She struggled with this decision and showed doubt about the moral foundation and consequences of the decision, especially for her faith:

My faith is important. Yeah, it is. It is. It is. It is. Yes. They never can take that away from me. No. I have my faith. I take my communion every week. I come to the church every week. And that's it. But I made that—that is a sin. I know an abortion is a sin. It was a sin. Yeah, in a way, yes. Yes. Because I'm not one to make a decision of having that child if it was already inside of my body, but that was the way I wanted it. I said, "God, please don't punish me." Every time I feel a pain, I said, "Oh, God, you're punishing me for what I did. Please don't!"

This conflict was a source of suffering for Camila. Spirituality and faith are therefore not conflict free but may actually be conflict-laden—coexisting with suffering and motivating agentic action. She prayed that God would not punish her for the decision she made. For Camila, the God of faith is a God whom she defines in terms of sin and punishment. She has a fear of God. This is an emotional condition that has been cultivated over time and has deep cultural significance.

Family and Social Life/Neighborhood and Relationship to Environment

The family has significance as a social structure in Camila's lived experience. The family is the central organizing unit of her social structure and is founded upon the relational Maternal home—a constituent of the Maternal Ground. The meaning of the family also has cultural significance and is rooted in Camila's early life experiences in the family home in her native country, living with her mother, father, and siblings. Camila acknowledges in her testimony that family life in her culture has a matriarchal structure. The mother is the head of the household. Camila assumes the Maternal role in this family structure after her mother's death. To some extent, she never abandons this family structure. It remains with her throughout her life.

Camila also understands the influence of neighborhood and community upon the social structure of the family. She describes her father's experiences after the loss of his wife and the loss of neighborhood and community support in his native island when he was transplanted to the States. Her father's health declined precipitously when this support was no longer available to him. He experienced his new environment as cold and unwelcoming. Camila's insight into the influence of neighborhood on health is also relevant to her own experience in the care facility. Her health and well-being are affected by her situatedness in the social structure of a family and the spatiality of a home that she has established for herself within the neighborhood environment of the care facility, which is itself a social system. These structures and systems of the environment have complex relationships to each other, to their respective constituents, and to the persons situated in the environment. The complexities of the care facility as a social system and its concomitant processes require consideration separate and apart from other social and cultural aspects of the environment because certain constituents of these systems and processes may lack intentionality and agency.

Second Temporal Moment: Vortex of Pain and Suffering

The study identifies pain and suffering as founded on the Maternal Ground. Pain and suffering are phenomenologically distinct constituents in the individual structure. Pain is not as salient in this individual structure as suffering. Suffering, however, does have salience. The study reveals that, for Camila, suffering is not contingent upon pain and can exist in the absence of pain. Camila undergoes pain and experiences suffering, even though she also experiences well-being. Certainly, when Camila first transitioned into the care facility, this was the case.

The trauma of disorientation experienced as the result of the loss of her husband, together with feelings of radical disorientation, dislocation, and displacement as the result of giving up her own home, are a source of suffering for Camila. She describes experiencing a deep depression after her husband's death and speaks explicitly in terms of her suffering. She describes this suffering as a sickness of the heart, not a physical illness. Although her family lovingly seeks her best interests in moving her to the care facility and although she passively consents, she experiences the loss of sociality and relationality, and a loss of role and functioning in the liminal state she finds herself in between worlds. The care facility has no qualities of life for her—eating, conversation, and going places. She experiences the move to the care facility as a kind of death in and of itself. For Camila, separation from family and home are among the core meanings of suffering. These core meanings have a deep cultural significance. The experience of suffering for Camila is a falling away from the state of well-being and happiness that she recalls in her past experiences. This state of well-being is rooted in the Maternal and its constituents, and the constituents are founded upon the Maternal structure. Spirituality stands out as being culturally significant in Camila's meaning of happiness. In the temporal moments revealed in this study, experiences of well-being and spirituality precede experiences of suffering. Suffering arises in the presence of spirituality. Camila speaks to this duality of lived experience:

> But the memories doesn't matter. I love baseball anyway. Oh, I love baseball. I was born in baseball in my house. My father, oh, yes. And my mother. Oh, we were Yankee fans. In [my native island]. We were Yankee fans. Yankee fans. We didn't have no television at that time. Just a radio. And we just used to—we used to sit down and listen to the baseball on the radio. And I remember all that, yes.
>
> Oh, I was young. Very young. I was about twelve years, eleven, twelve years old. Yes. And we used to go to the—my father used to take us to the horse races, the horse races, in [our native island]. And then after that, when I grew up, then I came to New York, I used to go to [the race track] with my husband. So I am into—the only thing I didn't learn was to drive, because he didn't want me to drive. He says no. Because he said that was for a man, a man's job. And no pants. He didn't want me to wear pants.
>
> He said, "That's not for you. That's for me. I am the man of the house. I wear the pants. You stay—" He used to say, "I wear the pants in the house. You wear the skirt, and you look much better for me." But he was a good guy. I don't regret anything. I feel satisfied. I had my trip to Europe, and I had a wonderful life. Really, I cannot regret it. It was good. I mean, they say that in life you have pains and aches. Pains and aches. And I had my pains and aches, but I had my wonderful time, too. Especially I had a good husband. He was good. He was wonderful. Yes. I think about him, yes. Yes, yes, yes, yes. I could never forget him. No. We used to work together. We used to go to work together in the morning and come in the evening.

Baseball bridges the old and the new worlds for Camila, and also the good and the bad in her experiences. She recalls her past experiences of baseball as a passion of her father's, as well as the love and happy memories of baseball, the races, going places in her native island, and the good experiences with her husband. But she also speaks of undergoing pain, and she holds the experience of undergoing pain and being well at the same time in her spatio-temporal horizon. Embedded in her horizon of experience is the desire to achieve the happiness that she recalls so richly from her past life now in her current situation in the care facility. As Camila recovers her sense of agency and is restored to a higher level of functioning in the care facility environment, she achieves an improved sense of overall health and well-being in her everyday activities and routines. But in her communications she continues to express experiences of deep loss of relational intimacy with family members who have died, with family members who are ill or estranged, and with other residents in the care facility. These losses are a severe contraction of her spatiality and temporality in the care facility environment, and a source of suffering for which she finds no immediate or long-term relief or comfort. Where at an earlier time she inhabited a space in which she was a competent worker with a good job who earned a salary; the head of a large family; and deeply loved by a mother, a father, and a husband—she now finds herself dwelling in a space in which her role is limited to being a good care facility resident and passively consenting to the love of family members who think they know what is best for her. In the episode with the resident who showed irreverence for her mother, Camila seemed to fail to live up to the expectations of what was required of the good care facility resident and sensed that she had disappointed not only the care facility staff but her family members. This was a source of anguish and distress for her. The losses of role, autonomy, control, and decision making—and the lack of access to culturally competent and sensitive health care and support—heighten Camila's sense of suffering and isolation.

Third Temporal Moment: Spiritual Well-Being, Resilience, and Recovery in the Face of Existential Suffering

Camila compellingly accounts for the coexistence and co-presence of an overall sense of well-being and general health, and experiences of pain and suffering. Camila speaks explicitly to this duality of lived experience. Camila has the capacity to simultaneously maintain conflicting and contradictory experiences. Undergoing experiences of pain and suffering do not completely disable her sense of agency or bar her achieving a sense of well-being. First, these are subjective determinations. They are not medical evaluations based upon physiological evidence, but multidimensional evaluations. Experiences of pain and suffering are fundamentally relational and have social and existential dimensions, as is evident in Camila's description of her husband's suffering and her understanding of his suffering experiences:

> He did suffer while he was ill. Oh yes, he did. He went to the radiation, and the doctors told me, "Miss [Name], he cannot tolerate the chemotherapy. It's better that we don't bother with that with him because it's too late. His cancer is going around the blood and everything. There's nothing we can do for him. He really have very little chance to live." Yeah. He was in pain, yes, all the time. They used to give him methadone. You know methadone, that they give to the drug addicts?
>
> And he didn't want the drug, and he said, "I have never been a drug addict. How come they give me that? They prescribe me that?" I said, "Listen, they say this is medicine, my dear. It's not you're going to be a cuckoo like this, the ones that are in the street, no. It's just that you need it for your pain. When you have the pain, you take the pill. Otherwise you have nothing to fear. You're not going to be addicted."

Camila's testimony conveys an overall sense of her well-being. She says repeatedly that she is "all right." She has accommodated to changes in her environment to a large extent and seems content. Her needs are being met, and she feels she is generally well taken care of. She is "going places," getting to see the world on her excursions out of the care facility, and has a room of her own. She has a walker to make it possible for her to ambulate wherever she wishes to take herself, and she is relatively autonomous in her activities of daily living. Her clinical state of health is the best that she feels it can be, and she is taking steps to monitor her own weight and blood pressure to the extent that she can to prevent exacerbation of her health conditions. Her family supports her and visits her regularly. She feels loved and wanted by them. She is supported by her nurse practitioner and her psychologist and can call upon her social worker when she needs her. She has at least one good friend among the residents (with whom she seems to be relationally oriented).

Decision Making

Camila shows variation in her attitudes toward end-of-life planning and end-of-life decision making, although overall there is an individual structure that emerges from the narrative data. She appears not to place great importance on future health care planning, but her conversations in that regard are more around formalistic, future health care planning than process-driven and relational conversations and communication. She is not focused on tools and documents. However, she understands the meaning and importance of treatment choices at the end of life and the deliberations and choices involved in forgoing care. These deliberations and choices are evidence of a practical agency at work in the present that involves evaluation of the problems at hand, characterizing the problems, and weighing the choices in context and the emotional significance of the choices.

Camila has consented to a Do Not Resuscitate Order, and she trusts her family members to make decisions for her when she is no longer able to make decisions for herself. She has taken time to have conversations with them about the end of her life. She describes the experience of her sister who is on a feeding tube and she expresses her desire not to have a feeding tube at the end of her life. What she says is that she enjoys the experience of eating and that she would not enjoy this type of medical feeding; it would be equivalent to being dead. She also describes the care she provided to her husband when he was dying and the help she gave him in understanding pain medication and relief of his pain symptoms.

Camila does not express a strong desire to participate in her own care planning meetings at the care facility. She seems to regard them generally as pro forma and as not having a big impact on her day-to-day care. But she does take an active role in managing her day-to-day care, inquiring actively of her nurse practitioner about her health status and actively monitoring her weight and blood pressure. She expresses a desire to avoid hospitalization, and when she does end up in the hospital on a nonemergency basis for a psychiatric evaluation, she critically evaluates the care in the hospital and the desirability of avoiding hospitalization.

Camila also has a very insightful understanding of the relationship between health, spiritual well-being, and end-of-life care, and her relationship to family, neighborhood, and environment. She demonstrates this understanding in her testimony about her father's suffering and end-of-life experiences, and her husband's end of life. Camila describes her husband as having a good end-of-life experience: as he was with his family and returned to his origins, to his native island. In bringing these past retentions to bear, Camila shapes her own intentionalities and desire about the meanings of a good dying experience that has the constituents of being relational and caring, and returning to one's origin through connectedness with family. Camila is engaged in a dynamic recovery from her suffering motivated by a desire and agentic drive for mobility, expanding spatiality, temporality, spirituality, and overall well-being. In the face of existential suffering, she displays remarkable resilience in all her intentionalities, enactments, and achievements in the world:

> No, I don't need assistance. I'm very independent here. I do my own washing. I do my own dressing, everything. I eat by myself. I have no—everything. I function like when I was 25 years old, thanks to God. I don't need nobody. I don't bother the nurses for nothing here, nothing at all. I make my own bed, I do everything.

Suffering, agency, spirituality, and well-being share space in Camila's life-world at the end of life, and are a part of her decision-making processes.

Conclusion

I looked forward to my visits with Camila when I would go to the care facility to interview my study participants. Camila was not like many of her peers in the facility because she was much more mobile, did not give the appearance of being weighed down by a heavy illness burden, and initially showed a good deal of confidence. This confidence was considerably shaken after the episode she recounted with her fellow resident concerning her violent response to invective she felt was leveled against her "mother"—really a cultural icon of the meaning "mother" had for Camila, rather than an idiom she did not understand. As a consequence of this conflict, Camila was sent for a psychiatric evaluation and was more closely monitored by the care facility thereafter. Afterwards, Camila communicated that she felt more threatened and less secure in the care facility environment. She was also humiliated when her family was told about the incident. Camila, even after being at the care facility for a number of years, continued to feel culturally isolated. Camila experienced this cultural isolation as a form of social suffering. These feelings of isolation were heightened by her reflective awareness of having violated her own cultural ethics in rejecting a traditional Maternal role by not having her own child. Camila's images of her loving husband, and his ongoing spiritual presence in her life, were the affordances that sustained her.

6 Suffering as Loss of Community

The Gifts of Grapes and Maternal Grace

One of the most delightful interviews I conducted during the course of my research investigations was with a "little sister" whom I shall call "Bernadette"—a very frail, 96-year-old member of a religious order of nuns, who resided in a care facility. She was dressed plainly but meticulously, and greeted me at the door of her room when I knocked with a hospitality and pleasantness that made me feel immediately welcome in her presence and in her home. Her freshness, mental acuity, and charm belied her ripe age and any suggestion that she was a care facility resident who might be struggling with illness, pain, or suffering. The interview began with Bernadette asking me about the purpose of the study and clarifying what questions she would be asked in the interview. I knew at that moment that the interview would take me to places not yet explored in my study of suffering.

After I explained that the focus of the interview was life-historical in focus, Bernadette shared with me the story of her coming to the care facility after a sudden illness and hospitalization, and her refusal to return to the assisted living facility where she had lived before. She described how unhappy she had been with the care at the previous residence, especially after she had developed a sudden illness and had not received the proper medical attention:

> Well, I was on—like I said, I was only there for three weeks. See, what happened was I got sick quite without any warning, very sudden, and not knowing the place, I was only there three weeks, you know, it was a big change from where I lived, you know, in the convent. It was our retirement house.
>
> And like, I didn't know any of the staff very well or anything. So, what happened was I got sick on a weekend morning. I went out to take a walk outside and all at once I started to shiver and shake and I had a temperature. And I didn't want to—I wanted to wait for the nurse to come when she returned. There was a nurse there but I had never seen her before, you know, so the other nurse I had contact with and I liked her very much. So when she came in the morning—see it was an assisted living place—and right away she said to me, "Well, I can't take care of you here." You know, "You have to go." So they sent me to [another] floor, which was really a rehab. It wasn't the

regular nursing floor, I understood later, and I was introduced to this nurse. And it was a man, a man nurse, a young man; he looked young to me. And so she said, "This is your nurse and he'll check on you." Well, I had a high temperature. I don't know whether I was delirious or not but actually, in one way, it was my fault. I didn't know enough to ring the bell they brought me that day. The way she talked he was going to check on me. Well, he never checked on me.

During that night—oh, it was a nightmare. I was so sick. And I didn't know what to do, you know. So, the next day they said they were going to send me to the hospital, which they did, and I was in the hospital two weeks. Then I wouldn't come back—I wouldn't go back there. I often wonder, I don't know whether I made a mistake or not because, after all, this is a [long term care] facility and that was an assisted living place where you have more freedom, you know, over—well, it's not the same thing. To start with, you know, I wasn't ready for [long term care]. Anyway, they were very kind to me here. I've been here now for five years.

Bernadette's decision not to return to the former residence was courageous: she received very heavy influence from her provincial not to make a change. The difficulty that Bernadette had with the decision was that many of her fellow sisters from the order to which she belonged resided in the past residence, and in deciding not to return there she knew she would suffer the loss of their community as she had known and enjoyed it. This was a sense of community to which she had grown accustomed in her years in the order, and living in the retirement community:

So, that's the only thing I missed, yes, not having, you know, someone to talk to, although I have a sister that visited me. Yes. And she took me out to the doctor's, you know. And so, and anything going on, they always came and picked me up. And we wound up doing a lot of our meetings together and everything at [name of assisted living residence]. They have a beautiful place on the ground floor. And that's where we, it's almost like our motherhouse now, you know, because we—our place, our retirement home is up for sale. It's been up for sale for number of years.

The Provincial wanted me to go back there. Yeah, because the—I'd be with the sisters. I mean, they'd had to come. I mean, I was separated from them so it always meant that somebody had to come and get me and then they had to send—the motherhouse, so they had to send a special communication. You know, it wasn't very convenient for the congregation. It would be easier for me to be at—and even the doctor, our doctor called me on the telephone and said why wouldn't I go back. I mean, it was a nice place.

The context Bernadette provided for her decision revealed that the decision she made was a conflicted one. Although she felt positively about the decision in light of her good health outcomes in the new facility, there was a pregnant pause in her reflections when she spoke about the loss of companionship and community. It was not at all clear that even with the efforts that she and the other sisters made to see to it that she was included in certain gatherings at the former residence, these efforts never quite made up for the separation and distance that she felt from the community on a day-to-day basis. There were residues of distress that were still evident in her emotional response to the decision, now unable to be undone.

These experiences of being separated from her community led back to her much earlier life when she first made the decision to enter the order. Unlike many of the other sisters who chose religious life in the early and middle part of the twentieth century, Bernadette entered the convent when she was in her late thirties. Before that she worked at the telephone company for 17 years. Her mother had become ill, and the nuns came to take care of her mother. She described how through the "grace of God" she made the connection with the Order:

> I never thought I was going to enter the convent. That's why I talk about the grace of God. The sisters took care of my mother. For about two—only about two weeks. The funny part was I never met the sister. Can you imagine that? We were keeping my mother home, my brother and I. We used to take turns from work. Taking time off from work. And I had just gone back to work and he was taking care of my mother. And I had a friend—it's a long story—I had a friend, she had rheumatoid arthritis. Did I tell you that story? Anyway, through her, she kept saying to me, "Why don't you call the sisters?" They were taking care of her. And then, "Get the sisters." Well, I really didn't want them. I had been educated by sisters. They were so fussy and all of this. I didn't want them. So they never came. I called and at first we had to call—in those days we had to call a priest or the doctor. And I called the priest and he called and they never called. So I never called [my friend] and told her. About three weeks went by and she called me, she says, "How are the sisters working out?" And I said, "They never came." She said, "Oh, they never came?" And I said, "No." Anyway, I called them. I called the priest in our parish. He happened to be the Vicar of Religious and he called them. The next day there was a sister there. My brother was home with my mother.
>
> Well, see, over time I had gotten more religious, you know, by going to mass and communion every morning. And I always say before she died my mother said something, "I'm going to storm heaven for you. You'll know when I get there." So she stormed heaven; she sure did. So that's why I was telling you about the grace of God. It's very difficult. How I had the nerve to go in the convent, the way I felt about sisters, that's the last place I wanted to be. But the call of God is really so strong that you can't, like I said to myself, I have to find out. I said "I have to find out if this is really what God wants of me." And I found out it was.

Once Bernadette entered the Order, she was sent for training as a nurse, and for many years visited the homes of families in the inner city where she provided care to those in need. She described the care as being more than simply medical or nursing, but tasks that involved supporting the family in sundry ways:

Yes, I was prepared for the work that I was going to do and I wanted to do it. That was the funny part. Like I said, there were times I was a little afraid, or not afraid but turned off by some of the places I went to, some of the things I saw. But I'm telling you, when God's work, when He wants something done, you know, it happens.

I wasn't shocked at some of the things I saw or heard, you know. I had more—if I was a young sister I might have, you know, been really—I had an understanding of family life.

I asked Bernadette a bit more about the history and the type of work that she did as a member of the Order:

Well, we're home nurses. Yes, [we make] home visits. Our focus was on the family. We were founded many years ago to keep the family together, mostly if the mother got sick. In those days people didn't go to the hospital like they do now. They were mostly cared for at home. And so we used to go and take care of the sick person. And then, actually, a lot of our work, we would then prepare meals and then do light washing, to keep the family together like so things wouldn't fall apart. So our focus has always been on the family.

And we never took any money, you know. We tried to go to poor people and working class, people who worked but, you know, didn't have much money. And so that work was very interesting, you know, going to different families. It was focused on the family.

Well, when our congregation was founded, he [the founder] said when you go into the home—see, he saw a need for it because he had a choir and the boys would be absent when their mother was sick. And so he said, he got a woman to help and he founded it and he said when you go into a home, you go for sickness, but there's always something else nine times out of ten that they need help with. So like I said, the focus was on if there were other problems with the children, anything. And of course, when he founded it, it wasn't like it is today but the sisters would, you know, as time went on we got social workers and we would have physical therapists and everything. But in those days, there was always something. Not only in those days, but as time went on, there was always something else, some other problem that we could help them with.

And we had—we used to have a meeting every month for the families, if they would want it we'd have a doctor or a priest or a nurse to speak, give a talk, and then we had refreshments. And we kept in contact with the family. And the sisters actually helped with these problems that they had, like often with children maybe, they needed help. Like we'd find out things that these people would tell sisters that they wouldn't tell other people, you know? Like, they trusted—they trusted sisters, you know? So, it's hard to put in words but we did, we did a lot unprofessionally, you know, because we weren't actually social workers. And then in the early days we weren't even nurses, but as time went on the congregation did send the sisters to be trained, mostly for nursing, but then as time went on for social work.

The work became very social, because we'd keep in touch with the families and their needs, you know. Lots of them were poor and they didn't know some things that they were eligible for as time went on. They didn't know. And it's hard to put in words, but we used to do everything, you know. And I often look back at some of the stories and I think how smart the sisters were, how they helped without any training.

I also asked Bernadette if her work resembled what is called palliative care and hospice today:

Yes. Yes, when people—we even would pass nights with them, to help the family get a rest. We'd stay there all night with the person, yes. We did—we took care of many dying persons. We would stay. They would be sick and as they—we'd take care of them. And then as they got worse or dying, we would stay at night. You know, it was—it's hard to explain, you know, what we did.

Bernadette shared that, after her hearing started to fail, she retired to the community house where the retired and infirm sisters lived, and there continued to provide care to her own sisters in the community. She described herself as still "agile" and well able to provide supportive care in this setting for the five years until it closed.

With this awareness of her life history, I asked her about her own experiences in the care facility where she currently resided, and those of her fellow residents. She described the difficult transition from the role of caregiver, especially in light of her life's work, to care recipient and patient:

Well, you know, it's hard to—it gets easier with time. When I first—what I find difficult, or did find, but I just, I have to be like a patient, is well, like medicine, for example. They give you medicine. They won't explain it to you and don't explain possible side effects.

Where I knew, at one time I used to know all the medicines and the side effects, but then now they don't tell you. And you can't ask questions.

It's those kind of things where I was used to knowing all the different things, like I'm trying to think of another thing besides medications. But to put it bluntly, you lose control when you come to a place like this. See, it's different in the assisted living place. You don't—you have more control and more freedom. But in a nursing facility, you're a patient and you're—you're a patient, period. I mean, you're not, they don't consult you about different things, you know, or you can't—it's—so that's hard. It's hard, in a way, to lose control, you know, of everything. Of course, with me, I've been more agile and I can walk and I can get around and all. People in wheelchairs, you know, are really, so it gets very hard for them. But even for me it was hard because being a nurse and knowing a lot of what goes into nursing and you see different things that you would do differently, you know, or you think that maybe they could have done more for the patient. Those kind of things are hard. That's what I say, that's with the control. And I'm a patient, too. So, if I—I've been sick several times.

I've been sick in bed at different times and having to depend on people coming in to, you know, if you ring them and they don't come right away, these kind of things, you know, are difficult.

Because after all, there are [several hundred] people in this facility. That's a lot of people. So there are things that you have to get used to. But outside of that, you get used to depending more on people. You have to. I mean, even going into it, going in the convent, I never thought I was going to be in a nursing facility. The sisters always took care of their own, you know.

Different people are, like different aides are kinder or they do more things for you, and even generally the whole place is kind. You know, you're taken care of.

Yes. If you're taken care of. That's why you're here. I mean, that's what one of the women that eats at my table, that's what she's always saying.

We're blessed. We're blessed because we're taken care of. Our needs are taken care of. Our beds are clean, maintained twice a week. And we get showers twice a week. That's another thing. You can't take your own shower. That's what I mean about a loss of control. But you get what you need so, and you're not—certain things you're not able to do yourself and so you have to accept it. You do have to accept it and that's not easy. But just like everything else, you have to be thankful because, as you get old, like one of my nieces sent me an article about a woman who is famous in her field for research on viruses. She was 94 and in her obituary her nephew said, "My aunt said people are living too long." And that's positively the truth. Because after a certain age, when you can't be an asset to society, you're dependent on people to take care of you. And it's gotten to be a big phenomenon. I mean, look at the hundreds of people here for care.

At first blush, Bernadette seems to have a positive attitude about all of the role changes she experienced in her transition to life in the care facility—from caregiver to care recipient, from one who made decisions to one for whom in many instances decisions are made, and from active engagement in the world to acceptance of dependency. Although she is grateful for the good care she receives, she also expresses some doubt about the value of living such a long life, with perhaps diminishing returns as dependency increases. In light of these reflections and her previous reflections about her decision to leave her community, it seems that Bernadette appreciates that it is her community that she values most and that its loss is a source of profound suffering for her.

In addition to the experiences of suffering that Bernadette described, such as loss of community and dependency, Bernadette describes the suffering she observed in other residents who were more dependent than she was in their basic life functions:

You know, one of the big things is wanting to go to the bathroom. Well, some people have to go to the bathroom so often. Now, in my day, when I was— they had catheters. They don't have, thank God, because people had lots of infections. But now they don't. They've done away with them, which is good. But the people sometimes have to go to the bathroom. You know, that's a big suffering that I feel for them, they're unable to go to the bathroom. I feel so bad. Yeah. It's hard... [long silence]. That's why I say you lose control of everything. But it's a—the life is a gift [to] the feeble. We cling to life regardless. You know, isn't that strange how people cling to life no matter what your condition is?

Bernadette is one of a subgroup of elderly women living in the care facility sites I visited who have devoted their lives to their orders and their mission. Two other residents also described the loss of community as a form of suffering they experienced in the transition to life in the care facility. These women presented as pillars of strength in the face of heavy illness burden and sometimes unbearable pain, and turned to their spirituality and faith to sustain them. For these women, the meaning that the Maternal has for them is living in community, and being engaged in relationships that are part of a social network. The dislocation from their community is a loss that is not dissimilar to the losses I heard described by other seriously ill elders in care facilities, such as the loss of a spouse or child, or even the loss of the home. The loss of community includes the constituents of the home and the relational dyad, but also includes multiple, nested and interlocking relationships that together constitute a highly integrated community for these members of religious orders. The members of the community share a common mission, abide by a set of governing rules, and are engaged in shared practices and shared decision making in ways that are uncommon in most social units, even the family.

Narrative of Virginia

My interview with a sister (whom I shall call "Virginia") who belonged to another religious order, and who was struggling with Parkinson's disease and chronic leg pain, as well as the transition to a radically altered life in a care facility as the result of her growing disabilities, was as inspiring and revealing in her testimony as Bernadette. In our first interview, Virginia engaged me in discussion about the St. Ignatian spiritual exercises and their revelatory purposes: guiding the process of self-discovery and becoming. Virginia also introduced me to the work of Thomas Merton (1966), *Raids on the Unspeakable*, and Merton's notion of the "Unspeakable" (p. 4)—the terrible things that are not visible and for which there are no words available to adequately describe them. In Merton's own words, he describes the "unspeakable":

It is the void that contradicts everything that is spoken even before the words are said; the void that gets into the language of public and official declarations at the very moment when they are pronounced, and makes them ring dead with the hollowness of the abyss. It is the … the emptiness of "the end." Not necessarily the end of the world, but a theological point of no return, a climax of absolute finality in refusal, in equivocation in disorder, in absurdity which can be broken open again to truth only by miracle, by the coming of God. Yet nowhere do you despair of this miracle.

(pp. 4–5)

It is in this broader context of the "Unspeakable", Virginia describes her response to learning of her diagnosis:

Yeah, you know, I think I'm pretty stupid, actually, because I didn't realize at the time how big a change that would make in my life, because there are people who have Parkinson's and you never even know it. So, I think it was more the sense of losing the community. Of course, I didn't and they'd be the first to tell me I didn't, but that's what it felt like, that I was being distanced by God from my community.

Well, I just knew that if God wants me here, or somehow in the eternal doings ... I think that it helps one to understand that we're part of something so much greater than ourselves and that we are loved. Otherwise, I don't think people could bear it. I know I couldn't. That the world is a difficult, difficult, horrendous place to be living.

Yes … and the "Unspeakable" is something within all human persons that is horrendously evil and can do evil things and can make evil decisions and all that kind of thing. So awful that Merton referred to it as the "Unspeakable," this thing inside of us, whatever it is, or surrounding us and fighting for our attention and all that. They don't name it anything or anything like that, but they just have the evidence of it; the horrendous things that normal, ordinary people, your next-door neighbors, would be involved in or that you might be involved in yourself.

All the different kinds of suffering in the world, yes, and the evil in the world. To know that we have enough for everybody, but what is it? Two-thirds of the world are terribly impoverished and suffering in anguish and civil wars here, there, and everywhere. These are the horrendous conditions of our world.

I think I thought it was part of God's—I don't want to say it was like a plan and every little thing. It's not that easy, but I believed it was not my choosing and that it came from the Lord and that because of the spirituality of finding God in all things, then anything I could do in this little room here in this facility is just as valuable to God as if I had these marvelous retreats all over the world and did them. In God's eyes, it's doing what God is inviting you to do to be part of the whole unfolding of the Divinity, you know? And that, in doing that, we are doing our vocation, so to speak and that this is what God wants of us and so on.

Virginia goes on to describe what she sees as the essence of living in community with other sisters, and what is lost in being displaced and coming to the care facility:

> A caring attitude, certainly, and understanding if you couldn't do all the things that you might like to do. Very generous. A few of us taught at places and we always were able to get a car signed out and the nitty-gritty things. People supported one another, yes. They all had the same desires in the sense of living out the spirituality. I feel I'm abbreviating it terribly and doing it a great disservice.
>
> The sister who usually drives me to the doctor, which is where I should have been this afternoon—here's the story: She called me yesterday; she fell and dislocated her shoulder, so she was calling to say she couldn't take me. I had to look around and there was no one really free to take me, so I had to cancel it.
>
> I think the people who are the most difficult to get through to are the aides, because they have the least training of anybody here in their field or whatever, if you can call it a field. For example, if we're in the dining room, let's say, they'll shout to each other across the room about, "Hey," something about bring this or bring that. It's just chilling on your nerves. They don't have any sense of decorum or anything. It's like, for example, if they're serving you soup, let's say and this is the soup bowl, they'll put their fingers all over the whole thing and then, throw it on the table like this. They don't have the common—
>
> There's something lacking there. When I look forward to what life may hold for me with Parkinson's in the future—which I know is a pretty bleak picture, what happens to a person for the most part—but when I think about it, the scene, the image I get is of being in the dining room with the aides feeding me. That's the image of hell. Yes, that's the picture, because I guess I've always been a little bit fanatical maybe about food and cleanliness and all that kind of thing. It's just something they don't share. It's sort of—I don't know.

In my second interview with Virginia, she shared with me that it is her experience that an older adult is either a resident or a non-resident in the care facility. In other words, she has found that there is very little fluidity in roles in the care facility. The resident is always a care recipient—and never a caregiver. Even as a member of the care facility resident council, Virginia felt powerless to effect any changes in the systems of care, though she found the staff very accommodating within the rigid social structure. She lamented the absence of reciprocity in relationships or any meaningful communication in the care facility life:

> I was thinking again of the dining room. Now, I'm at a table in the dining room with two other sisters, okay? One of them never, never speaks. I think she's partly deaf, but I can't really tell. But anyway, she never, never speaks,

but now I've gotten her to the point where she'll be laughing. She'll take part in things. I bring her little treats when no one is looking, stuff like—she's 92, so she loves that. She's coming along.

Then, the other sister who sits with us has some kind of a problem. I don't know what the problem basically is, but she spits out all her food. It's very disgusting to look at, like she spits it out all over herself and it flies across the table sometimes, too. Then, the third one is very, very sick and I expect any day to hear that she had died. Now, that's the table. So, as far as being able to talk with someone, there's no one.

Virginia's accounts reveal the depth of her spiritual suffering beyond any suffering associated with disease process. In trying to understand better what she was experiencing, I asked her if she was struggling with a loss of meaning. Our gazes met—she did not shrink from wanting to faithfully respond to my question—and she said no, her struggle was not about meaning at all:

But do you remember when Mother Teresa died, that her journals were printed?

It said how she had experienced the desert all this time in her life. Did you read about that?

A feeling of depression, of emptiness, of nothingness, of all of that.

It's sort of like your feelings. Your feelings go wacky. You feel depression, but the spiritual teaching is that in that very depression or in that very darkness or in that nighttime that you experience, you will find the Resurrection. The Cross leads to the Resurrection, that kind of thing.

No. I have all the meaning in the world. That's what keeps me going is the meaning of it all, I really do believe.

It's more like an emptiness. Yeah, an emptiness, a depression.

Yes, and I have no idea what it is and I don't feel it as a joy or anything, but you know, at the Easter vigil, which is such a magnificent thing—in a sense, it's the spiritual exercises compressed—but anyway, in the Easter Liturgy, the one at night at 12:00 at night where they sing The Exultet? That's where it talks about the night and it says how, "O, night, more beauteous than the dawn." It has all these wonderful things about the night. Well, what you feel is the night, but what you believe is beyond the light.

[I feel the night], I do. I do. I feel the loneliness, yeah. But it's like nothing you could correct or anything. It's just that's how life is.

Or maybe part of the emptiness is that you don't have any emotions anymore. You just have your faith to hold onto. If you didn't believe, you'd have nothing. There'd be no reason to go on living, really.

If you didn't have your faith, but I mean, the right kind of faith. Faith that's knowing and loving God. Knowing we're loved, that kind of faith.

When I left Virginia, I carried with me the overpowering image of the "Unspeakable" in thinking about elders' experiences of suffering. I realized, too, that it was I who was the receiver of grace in my interview with Virginia, as in so many others.

Narrative of Josephina: Diverse Communities

In the care facility setting, there are many types of communities that are present even among residents who are not members of formally organized religious orders. The care facility itself may be viewed as a community, but in its midst there are sub-communities. For example, residents may form alliances that are a source of the Maternal care lacking in the system or community as a whole. "Josephina," a 93-year-old female in the long-term care unit of a care facility, is an example of one elderly resident who struggled with a heavy illness burden, yet turned to her fellow residents for the type of Maternal care she did not always receive from the care facility staff. Like Angelique and Camila, she also assumed the role of caregiver, in the context of her own family life, from within the walls of the care facility.

Josephina was admitted to the care facility well over five years ago. She has a daughter, granddaughter, and great-grandson, as well as nieces—but they were not able to visit regularly. She maintained regular contact with them by phone. She had hypertension and chronic kidney disease, as well as congestive heart failure, diabetes, atrial fibrillation, moderate depression, edema, anemia, and dyspnea. She was wheelchair-bound and required assistance with ambulation and activities of daily living, but had been evaluated as having no pain. Josephina was eager to speak with me when I came to visit her, and over a period of several months I was able to capture her narrative voice.

Josephina describes her roots in the Maternal dimensions of existence in her country of origin, and the relational intimacy she shared with her mother, whom she lost to cancer, and other family members:

> My mother died very young. She had cancer. About 62 or something like that. Yeah.
>
> Oh, yeah she suffered a lot. At that time, they didn't even know what it was until a long time they found out. Something in her throat. And she didn't smoke. Oh, yeah, it was hard on my sisters and myself. I was 21. And I had a younger brother. He was 17.
>
> And I had another older brother who was born here. I had a sister and a brother who were born here. I was born in [Europe]. No, I wasn't born in this country. I was born near [a city in Europe] somewhere. Oh, we came over when I was young. I was six or seven. I had all my schooling here in this country. Oh, yeah, my mother married in [Europe]. But then they came here. And then there was the Spanish influenza, and she lost the two children.
>
> She suffered. She must have had nine. We were six, and she lost a few.

From the outset, illness, loss, suffering and spirituality are core meanings of Maternal and relational intimacy experiences for Josephina. She describes her mother's suffering in losing two of her children and dealing with terminal illness, and she communicates a strong sense of being empathically, spiritually, and relationally connected with her mother and her siblings in her mother's suffering condition.

Prior to these experiences of shared suffering, however, Josephina's experience of relational intimacy is formed upon a Maternal Ground of care and nourishment. This care involves being housed, fed, touched, and profoundly loved in a pre-reflective, holding environment. Josephina describes being immersed in these meanings of Maternal loving care, nurture, and support that she in turn provides to her own family in her adult life:

> My daughter was brought up Catholic. She went to Catholic school. Although my husband had died already; he died so young. About 40. Not even 40. He had a heart attack. And she was about five, I think. Yeah, she was young. And I brought her up by myself. Yes, she was my only child. Oh, yeah, I brought her up myself. I went to work. And my sister took care of her. My niece's mother, her mother Rose. Yeah, Rose took care of my daughter. Well, they lived—we lived all in the same neighborhood. I lived in the [the city], but then when I lost my husband, I moved to [another part of city], where my sisters were. Yeah, so I could be near them. So I got a lot of help from them. I sewed in the neighborhood. We made gowns. Yeah, in the neighborhood, though. It was one block I walked to go to work. Yeah. It was very good. That's why I worked till 75 years old. Yeah. Because to me, it was in the same place. Yeah, I had good benefits. Yeah, I had health benefits. And death benefits. Well, yeah, I had a pension and retirement benefits. We got that.
>
> And that's the way I lived. And we got along very good. Oh, yeah. I would have worked even more if my daughter didn't need help and I went to live with her. She needed me. Always. Always. Her husband died, too, very young. He was about 37. And she's a widow, too. Oh, yeah she was struggling. And then there's a mother-in-law problem and a lot of things going on. Oh, always supportive. Always. I wish I could do more. Oh, I wish I could do more. It is hard for me. Because we only get $50 a month here, and when she needs it, I give it to her.

The descriptions of Josephina's early widowhood and role in raising her daughter by herself and her continuation of that role in her end-of-life illness show the relationship of the Maternal dimensions of existence and their structure across Josephina's lifespan to her current place in the care facility. Josephina's experience of the Maternal is fundamentally social and relational. She relied on her sister and her community to support her in her Maternal role as a single mother. She also relied on her role as a wage-earner and a producer in the community, through which she accrued social and economic benefits. These benefits helped to sustain her provision of care and nourishment to her family.

Losses of Maternal foundations and ground of relational communication

Later in her lifespan, Josephina turns to her daughter for care after she suffers a stroke and becomes dependent. She experiences multiple losses of the constituents of the Maternal when her daughter can no longer take care of her:

> I went home after therapy at the first. And they sent me home.
>
> Yeah. I was in outpatient for therapy. And then they… my daughter suffers with her knees and all. She couldn't take care of me. So, I mean, it was too much for her. Yes, I was living with my daughter at the time. And that's what it worked out, that she had to call the ambulance and they took me back here. I lost my voice. It changed. It got groggy. But I could always talk. I had my— thank God, I had my senses yet.
>
> Well, she spoke to me. She says, "Ma, I can't do it anymore." So I suggested they send me back and try again. So I'm here since then. Yeah, just about here five years. I gave up my place. Well, I didn't mind giving up my place because I had my grandchildren. So I was happy to move. But it didn't work out. The rent was too high. Oh, the rent was $140, something like that. It was high. So we couldn't get—we couldn't—No, we couldn't stay there.
>
> We moved to a place, to a smaller place, together. And before you know it, I got the stroke. I don't know why. I used to walk so much. No, we didn't come here together. Then I had to come here. She couldn't take care of me no more. She suffers with sciatica and with bad legs. No, she couldn't take care of me anymore. She tried. And so I transferred here from home. No, she couldn't take care of me. She's almost 60.

Josephina experiences her stroke and separation from her daughter as a kind of shock—a sudden and unexpected displacement. While at first she receives therapy at home, she ultimately ends up going to the care facility when her daughter tells her she can no longer take care of her. Josephina experiences this as a compounding of the shock. She has retained her faculties, but sustained deeper losses that she is still struggling with five years later—losses of home and sense of well-being, care and relational intimacy with her daughter and family in the home, and independence and autonomy in functioning. She becomes dependent and alludes to losing her voice. While she maintains that she was able to talk, there is the beginning of a thread about voicelessness that she describes in more depth in the context of her situatedness and shrunken spatiality and temporality in the care facility:

> Because I have no voice and I call people, they don't hear me. And so, she's [her roommate] my voice otherwise. She'll call for me.
>
> Or if I can't get to my bell, she'll ring for me, you know. We get along all right. Only we wish we had—I had more room because I just have a space where I could sit there and I have to wait.

The relationship between relationality and communication is profound. As Josephina experiences losses of sociality and relationality with family and community, she also loses the relational intimacy that is the ground of meaningful communication. Relationality founds communication, and the loss of relationality diminishes access to and opportunities for communication with relational others.

Generous Maternal praxes and vocational project of care

Josephina's generous Maternal praxes survive her illness and disabilities in her frail, seriously ill state. She continues her supportive role in manifest and non-manifest ways from her wheelchair:

> I am always supportive of my daughter. I wish I could do more for her. Oh, I wish I could do more. It is hard for me. Because we only get $50 a month here, and when she needs it, I give it to her.

There are two essential constituents of Maternal care that emerge in her testimony: goodness, and moral and ethical responsibility. Josephina takes up her Maternal role in light of the aim of producing good. Her only interest is in assuring the well-being of her daughter and her family. Her vocational project is caring for them, even in her limited capacity as a wheelchair-bound, disabled, and frail individual. But her capacities as an agent are not limited by physical infirmities. She has strong desires and spiritual intentionalities to be relationally connected with her daughter and her family, and her testimony describes her enactments to fulfill the meanings of her intentions to bring happiness and flourishing to her family.

Home as dwelling, inhabiting, welcoming hospitality, protective environment, nourishment, and origin

An essential constituent of the Maternal Ground is the home: the place in which the elder person dwells. In all of Josephina's statements, there is evidence of the home emerging as a salient constituent in her experience. Josephina speaks about her home as origin—where she was born and where she came from, cradled in the Maternal relation. The welcoming hospitality and protective environment of the Maternal womb and Maternal cradling are the origin of experience, nourishment, and contact with body, self, and the world. A sense of well-being arises in the dwelling of the Maternal home-place. Losses of dwelling and sense of well-being are what create displacement for Josephina when she has to give up her home and the home she shared with her daughter.

But the Maternal home-place as origin is also the origin of a horizon of experience with limitless possibilities. The home in this sense is inhabited and is a place of generativity. Josephina always adopts an agentic stance of inhabiting even after she has given up her home and is situated in the care facility. She expands her spatiality and temporality in the care facility through this stance toward the world and an attitude of praxis. She speaks of always being supportive of her daughter. She inhabits her daughter's world, experiences and challenges. What she means is that she aims to be supportive of her daughter in light of producing good. The intentionality of her action is to help her daughter by providing emotional and financial support.

Desire and agency

Desire and agency are also essential constituents of the Maternal Ground. Desire is a movement of intentionality that is emotional in character. Agency is rooted in desire and involves temporal enactments of intentionality. Josephina's testimony reveals many desires and many agentic processes—including the desire to walk, to be relational, to be free of pain, to feel better. She expresses a desire to walk even in her declining functioning:

> I do walk. They take me for a walk. I walk about 50 feet and that's it. On the floor, yes. With help, of course. Not alone. Yes, with the physical therapist. I walk almost every day. I think she has one day off, or something. And that's nice. But I get very tired.

Josephina experiences misery and burden because of being wheelchair-bound and dependent, constantly waiting to be taken care of by others in order to have her basic needs met. Her desire to walk transcends her burden, even though she realizes that she will never be able to regain full capacity to ambulate as a result of the stroke she suffered. The walking that she does do with the physical therapist is goal-directed, an agentic process and praxis. The fifty feet she walks is an achievement for Josephina in the course of her long day.

Josephina also has a desire for sociality and relationality that manifests itself in a number of different ways. She likes going places and participating in the recreational activities in the care facility and outside the care facility:

> Tonight we're having a dinner and dance. At five o'clock, we're going down to the auditorium and we're going to have dinner, and whoever can dance will dance. We have music. It's nice.
>
> We make up poems and stuff like that. Oh, yes, I do enjoy that. And sometimes I go where they paint. I try to be a painter. Oh, I try to keep myself going. I don't want to just sit there. So we play bingo, and sometimes there's the aide that comes and we play games.
>
> But a [the recreational therapist], who's the head of the—she takes care of the—what would you call it? Anyway, she takes care of the program of the floor. She's been on vacation for about three weeks, but she's coming back Wednesday, and I'm so happy. Because there's more going on when she's there. And that's what makes me happy. She's coming back. Oh, yes, I do have a good relationship with her. She's so—oh, good God, I did miss her. She's such a wonderful person!

I try to go everywhere. I went to the ballgame, the Yankees in the new ball park.

Oh, I loved it. I loved it. And they won that day. It was very thrilling. And sometimes I go to the casino in Yonkers. I have been places where I never went to before. But I loved it. And even the casino, we used to go to Jersey then. I manage because they place us in special places, where the chairs go, where the group goes, whatever. When I'm out, it's not too bad; I don't think about the swelling in my legs. I feel good when I go out and sometimes we go to Kmart, shopping. They do a lot of things. Right, it takes my mind off the suffering. And we have gardening here; we planted the flowers here, which is good.

While the giving up of her own dwelling that she shared with her daughter was a deep and traumatic loss, Josephina conveys a positive outlook and general sense of well-being, and expands her spatiality in the care facility by going places and participating in activities. This is another form of agency and praxis. Her chronic condition of edema, however, is a constraint on her activities and outward movement into the world.

Josephina's most powerful activation of desire and self-agency is her persistence in trying to reach her daughter when her phone is broken, and the continual engagement of her projective capacities to fashion a futural horizon for her daughter and her family:

No, while the phone was broken I didn't speak to my daughter, but she used to call. She called the desk, you know, and I talked to her a few times there. She knew what was going on. My daughter is living in a—what do you call those homes? She hasn't got an apartment. She's waiting for them to give her an apartment. She's in a shelter there, in the city. Well, as long as I talk to her. Of course I'm worried, because my granddaughter lives with her. She's there, too, with the baby. There are three of them. And they're just waiting for an apartment. Where do they put her? In Brooklyn.

She's far away, but she always lived in the Bronx. And that's the bad part.

Oh, sure, I'm a little worried about her. She's got bad knees, she can't walk so good. She's not well now. No, no, she has a lot of pains in the knees. She has to use a cane. Sure, she uses a cane. She's probably almost disabled—and now there's a baby, and she's involved with the child. My daughter. Otherwise, she could be working, you know. But she's 59. She lives with her, her daughter. Yes, in the shelter. They're together. Yeah, that's good, that they're together. But still, it would be nice if they had their own place. No, she's not that fit to come to see me. If she lived closer, you know, but from Brooklyn, no. My granddaughter came. She came more than once. She brought the baby. But, you know, it's a hard trip to take.

And she's got, I think how old is he? 16 months? I talk to him on the phone—well, make noises, anyway. But he repeated "Nana." He repeated that once, and I couldn't get him to say it again. But he's pretty smart. They used to come often, when they lived in the Bronx. But she had trouble with her in-laws. She lived there and she had to get out. Terrible. Of course, very hard, not being able to see them more often. You know, I'd like to see them. Because I'm 93 years old.

At 93, Josephina actively inhabits the Maternal role from her wheelchair in the care facility. Josephina's relationship with her daughter is very meaningful to her, and being separated from her daughter is a source of suffering. When her phone was broken, she could not reach her daughter; this was a primary form of communication for her—a way of relational access to a significant person in her life. The Maternal relation has meaning in Josephina's end-of-life illness experience. Even disabled as she is by chronic conditions and persistent pain, she has a desire to be in a Maternal relation with her daughter and a strong sense of agency in the Maternal role. Josephina's testimony reveals the important founding relationship between the structures of relationality and communication in lived experience. The Maternal Ground founds desire for relational communication. Josephina not only actively worries about the welfare of her daughter, her granddaughter, and great-grandson, but actively engages in goal-directed, projective thinking and imagining about her daughter's future and that of her family. Where will they live? How will they take care of themselves? She understands the gravity of their situation and the urgency of their needs. This activity is a type of agency even though it may not be as conspicuous as the praxes of eating and walking.

Ethical relation and moral agency

The relation between Josephina and her daughter is defined by the moral claims embedded in and originating in the Maternal Ground. Josephina has a primary responsibility of care for her daughter and her daughter's well-being, and it is a responsibility that is not abnegated or vitiated by her existential suffering condition:

> Of course, my main worry is my daughter, her well-being, and my granddaughter. And my grandson, I have a grandson and a granddaughter. And we wish, we hope, that everything comes out all right.

Josephina is connected and reconnected to her daughter's world through the telephone. It is her lifeline to sociality and relationality. And her primary relational connection in this primal moment in the horizon of her experience is the Maternal relation with her daughter and granddaughter. Although their visits in person are infrequent, she maintains a relational intimacy with them by communicating with them by phone. She tries to speak with them every day and she says she loves talking to them. The love, worry, and hope she describes are complex emotions that disclose the values she attaches to the relationships she has with her family. These are closely held relational attachments in which she invests all of her trust, fidelity, and obligation. The Maternal relation in which Josephina stands to her daughter is an ethical relation. Josephina's intentionalities and aims in light of her daughter's needs, reveal the moral claims that her daughter and her family make upon Josephina—and Josephina's enactments and responses as a moral agent. The Maternal Ground and Maternal relation is a primary domain of moral experience for Josephina.

Faith and spirituality

Faith and spirituality are essential constituents of Jospehina's individual structure of suffering. These dimensions of the individual structure do not have as much salience in the narrative data as other constituents of her experience that are more visible, but their presence is made prominent in Josephina's testimony. Their less salient presence needs to be attended to in an explicit way to make visible how these structures are operating in the overall individual structure.

In her first two statements above, Josephina describes her early life experiences in the Maternal relation in her place of origin, and also her adult life experiences establishing a home for her daughter. Both of these experiences are laden with spiritual intentionalities and meaning. The Maternal relation is not reducible to a bodily state of being, but has existential and spiritual dimensions. Josephina's spiritual intentionalities arise in the context of the Maternal ethical relation dynamically enacted in Josephina's relation with her daughter. The ground of moral obligation in this ethical relation is the call of the other and substitution of the other for the self.

Pain and suffering

Josephina experiences a very heavy burden as a result of her chronic illnesses and health conditions. She has congestive heart failure and is in chronic, persistent discomfort and pain with edema in her legs. She is also in chronic discomfort because of the diuretics she is taking for edema and other medications for chronic conditions. Josephina's persistent and unabated pain is clear. Although she receives medications, she seems to have no real relief for her pain. There is evidence that the medications in some instances heighten Josephina's pain. Josephina's experiences of pain are multidimensional—experienced bodily, but also beyond the physical and the bodily experience. There are emotional aspects of the pain experience that are apprehended by others. Josephina's pain burden has existential dimensions that are sometimes intolerable and lead to suffering. Josephina describes both the temporality of her everyday discomfort and the extent of the burden imposed by her chronic conditions:

> Well, there are days where I've been good and there are days when not so good.
> Yes, see I have—I got a stroke and this leg is still bothering me. Yes, it's causing me a lot of discomfort. Especially at night. As it gets later, you know.

My foot swells. And it hurts underneath. And they know that. The nurses know that. I wear special socks, which are tighter than—oh, God! I think that I am in discomfort most of the time. Yeah. No, I don't get much relief.

The socks that Josephina wears for her edematous condition emerge in the narrative data as salient evidence of her pain. She describes the socks in detail, and the ordinary way in which their rolling down her adipose legs heightens her bodily pain and cultivates in her intense feelings and emotional responses to her pain:

> But I suffer with these legs a lot. My legs are my major concern, right?
>
> No, my legs don't pain. The socks pain. I'm always asking for socks, which they don't send me. Because I wear special socks. Well, I would have been better if I didn't have to wear these long socks, and they don't give me any more. And they come up to here. You see, they form a roll. They roll. You can feel it, a roll, you know, and they get tighter and tighter. And after about this time, my feet feel like they're paralyzed or something. They're specially just for—this is where I had my stroke. And it seems at this time, almost always the same time, I'll have to go to the bathroom. So. And I have to wait for somebody to go because they don't allow me to go alone. But I could go alone if I want to. I manage. But I have to wait. Oh, God. They don't feel so—they take all their time.
>
> Yes, I find it hard. Being in the chair. Oh, yeah. Very. Because these socks, too, they hurt after an hour or so. After this hour, they hurt me. And I still have to go down to eat because I eat downstairs, and come up. And then by the time they come and put me to bed, I mean—that's why I go to bed early. Sure, because I have to keep my feet up.

In her situation, Josephina experiences something as ordinary as a pair of socks as a heavy pain burden. She repeatedly makes reference in her testimony to the socks—medical socks—that she is given to wear to help keep the swelling down in her legs. There is no evidence in the narrative data of any conversation with any members of the health care team surrounding Josephina's experience of this burden or what it means to her. She has been evaluated as having no pain. The meaning of the socks for Josephina is very significant in her everyday lived experiences in the care facility—negotiating her chronic conditions and doing the best she can as a good resident and citizen "of the community". This is part of her effective agency.

Josephina also demonstrates emotional responses to her pain burden that have been cultivated over time and disclose the negative values she attaches to her pain experiences. She expresses feelings in response to her pain—bodily feelings of being paralyzed, and feelings of anguish that underlie her cultivated emotional response of negatively valuing her situation as burdensome. These narratives help to illuminate the various constituents of the pain experience—the sensory, cognitive, and emotional dimensions of pain. But Josephina's pain is also relational, social, and existential in its dimensions. Others, such as the care facility staff, apprehend her pain experiences in her situatedness in the care facility and her emotional responses to her pain:

> Well, I've had my good days and my bad. Because I suffer with this foot a lot. With my foot. It swells up, especially this one. Yes, the left one. Because I had the stroke. And sometimes, it's very painful until I go to bed, and they take it off. I try to tell them to put me in bed earlier, so they could take off my socks. And I eat upstairs. That's what I do. And I shower. When they shower me early and they put me to bed. And I eat in my bed. They bring the food up because I eat here. And I eat there. And so every time they take off my socks, which are horrible. But now she tried new—
>
> Yes. It hurts, especially onto this foot. Yeah, the left one. And it's a horrible feeling. And I hate to be in pain. Well, yeah, I'm in pain. Sometimes it starts earlier, and sometimes it starts a little later. Today, right now, they're not so bad because these are new socks she's trying, and I hope they work.
>
> Yeah. She gave me new socks, so, I don't know. It's not so bad as other days.
>
> Oh, yeah, some days are better. It's according to the weather, because if it's very hot, they swell more, see. And they hurt.
>
> Oh, they give me Tylenol. It doesn't do much good. Not for that pain. No, it doesn't control the pain. But you have to take what they give you. Well, I talked to R. [staff nurse] yesterday about something stronger. He's the nurse. And if he's on tonight, maybe he'll give me something stronger. Well, he has to report it and make papers. They don't just give them out. Oh, yeah. He knows I'm in pain.

The social and relational dimensions of the pain experience stand out. "He knows I'm in pain," Josephina says of the staff nurse. This is a powerful description of others' access to the pain experience, apprehension of what the suffering person is going through, and the suffering person's emotional response to the pain she is undergoing. But the dimensions of the pain experience go beyond the social and relational to the whole existential condition. Josephina has a low sense of agency about whether she can make any change in her circumstances. "You have to take what they give you." She feels powerless, yet she transcends this powerlessness and asks for a change in the medication to control her pain. She has a good relationship with the staff nurse, and she communicates with him about what she needs.

Josephina makes it clear that she desires relief from pain and wants pain medication—whether sleeping pills or pain medications. This is part of her agentic process—directing her agency toward medical decision making that will bring relief of her pain:

> If it didn't pain me at night, I wouldn't even think about it.
>
> A little at night when I first take them off, they sort of—ache, right.

If I want to get pain medication, yes. Oh, I get a sleeping pill. Yes, yeah, I sleep.

I suppose I wouldn't sleep all night without a sleeping pill because it's been done where they forgot to give it to me or something. I'm up all night. I don't sleep.

I have to have it. I used to take a sleeping pill when I was well, and I was home. I took sleeping pills. And now I still need them. And they give me, but only they changed it. They give me Ambien. They call them Ambien but they're generic. So it takes me a little more time to fall asleep. But I sleep. Yes. I finally sleep, I know.

Suffering

Like pain, suffering is also social and relational—and multidimensional—in nature. However, suffering can exist without pain. Pain is not an essential constituent of suffering. Pain can be a bodily form of suffering that becomes intolerable and can lead to suffering. There are multiple sources of suffering for Josephina—loss of sociality and relationality, loss of the home, loss of a loved one, loss of control, assaults on personal dignity. An accumulation of these experiences rises to the level of existential suffering:

Yes. That's the worst thing asking people do to things for me. You have to depend on somebody. And some of them, they're not nice about it, either.

She comes and I tell her, "I got to go." "You went once, I'll take you one more time. If you have to go again...." I don't know. It's very hard sometimes.

And yet some of them are so nice. They take you anytime you need to go. And they change nurse's aides. I don't always have the same aide. I have an aide who's there most of the week, but he's a man. And I have to take him because they used to have different nurses. I had one, and my roommate had one. But now they put one nurse to each room. So she happened to have a male. So I have to take him. But it don't bother me because I'm too old to think of anything about a man.

See, the foot swells up. And then I guess my toes hit the shoe. And there's I get the pain.

It's the stroke. No, I can't take care of it myself. I can't move this leg. I mean, I move it very little. And I walk. I could walk with this leg with the walker and with an aide, of course. And I walk about 50 feet, and that's—I do it every day.

She comes every day.

I wish I could do more and more, but I can't. Maybe a little miracle someday, I'll start to walk again. Oh, yes. I do believe in miracles. But well, I could only wish. Because they don't happen all of a sudden. And that's the story of my life. And I don't know why I got a stroke because I walked miles. I did a lot of walking. And it still didn't help, I guess. I guess when it has to be, it will be.

I don't have control. I don't know—yeah, I feel very dependent. And I hate that. I was wishing that I just could do everything myself so I wouldn't mind sitting here. But don't forget, I sit about 12 hours a day. I get up at 6:00 A.M. And I sit in this chair. Until she comes and I do walk. Oh, it's very long sometimes. Right.

Well, I'm trying to control it.

I tried many things. This leg is pretty good. I don't have trouble with this leg, but this one, say, I could just go that much and that's all.

Josephina speaks to her state of dependency and everything that she experiences in this state of dependency. One significant part of her experience is being forced to rely on others to take her to the bathroom, and the indignities she is subjected to sometimes as a result—such as Bernadette describes. This is a significant custodial need because of her edematous condition. She describes having to wait for long periods of time before having her needs met, and of sometimes being treated in a demeaning fashion by care facility staff. Waiting imposes a heavy burden on Josephina. Thus, in addition to the limitations on activities of daily living that she experiences, such as toileting, she experiences continuous assaults on her dignity and personhood. She links these negative relational experiences to staff turnover at the care facility, another relational loss. She says she doesn't always have the same aide assigned to her. Josephina is unable to establish trusting relationships with the aides upon whom she relies for care. These multiple losses of personal dignity, agency, and trusting relations with staff clearly heighten the distress associated with Josephina's loss of functioning and dependency due to her edema and stroke conditions.

The accumulation of burden, however, does not end here. Josephina loses her friend in the care facility and is kept away from her friend's services because of her bowel condition:

Yeah, I feel alone. I feel very alone. And I have this leg that I can't move. And they have to take me to the bathroom, and I hate that. I like to go myself. Oh, some days, they don't put on the—I have special socks, and they don't put them on right. They put them on loose. They make rings around my fat thighs. Yes, it does cause a lot of discomfort. Until I get to bed. Then I feel better. Yeah. That discomfort is what it is.

And I walk every morning. Yes, with the physical therapist. And I walk about 50 feet or something. Yeah, every day. And that's my exercise. Oh, I like it. But what keeps me back—I could do more—is this arm's weak. Yeah, the left side is weak. And I have to put my pressure all mostly on the right hand. And I get tired. But otherwise, I'd do better.

Oh, yeah they had something here to honor my friend who passed on. We'll have a memorial, I'm sure. We write a poem about her. We each say what we thought. And they read it down with the father. Oh, yeah. We did start working on the poem.

Well, not that she was only a friend of mine, but—maybe this sounds funny—but every day, I used to have little goodies that I used to give to her. She loves grapes, and I always brought her—we got—I eat downstairs, and sometimes I'd give her something different. And grapes she loved. Oh, and I always brought the grapes up to her. No, no she didn't go downstairs to eat.

Well, she has something with her leg, too. But she walked good. I mean, with the aid of the—with her aide there, she walked very good. In fact, she walked better than me. And she was doing so well, you know. Then bang, it was like an explosion.

Oh, my mate broke the news, the one that—E. [roommate]. She waited for me after lunch. She eats up here, see. I eat downstairs. But then I come up, and I stay in the hall. And she waited for me outside, and she broke the news. They found her in the morning. I think when they came to give her the exercise.

And they found her. She didn't know she was dead, but she looked different. And then they called the nurses and all that, and they went in and they pronounced her dead. And they came to take her. And they're having a service somewhere. I can't go because I can't walk, and I have trouble with my bowels. They give me certain pills to make me go all the time. And if I have to go there, it's too much. That's why sometimes I keep back from going someplace because I'm afraid of my bowels. I don't know. I don't know if I should take those pills.

They give me iron because I'm a diabetic, and I'm anemic. You wouldn't believe it. That's what they say, anyway. And they give me these iron pills, and they constipate me, and I have a lot of trouble. And they don't—they like— they take you to the bathroom. You go once, and they—to them, it's a lot. And sometimes, I suffer with my... I have to wait. Oh, yeah, I'm in a great deal of discomfort. No, I'm not happy with these pills. No. I think I'm going to stop them myself and see what happens. Yes, it [the pill] does cause discomfort.

So now, I used to give her my banana every day. Yeah. Once in a while, I'll eat one. And I used to—I says, "Here," and I used to roll myself over there if they're eating, and I gave her the banana.

The convergence of Josephina's experiences of struggling with the limitations of her chronic conditions and the effects of her medications, the loss of her friend, and her increasing isolation deepen insight into the core meanings of existential suffering for a 93-year-old woman confined to a wheelchair in a care facility. Josephina is immersed in misery, distress, and discomfort. She is in constant discomfort because of her bodily functions, and her medications sometimes heighten this discomfort and further constrain her activities and expansion of spatiality. It is a terrible sorrow that she cannot even attend her friend's funeral because of her loss of control of bodily functions. Her dwelling space in the care facility continues to shrink as she loses her dearest friend and her relational intimacy, and her opportunities for forming new relationships with other residents are minimal, as the frailty of the other residents makes them also vulnerable to serious illness and demise. She has few trusting relationships with professional staff, and losses of sociality and relationality extend to Josephina's limited access to her daughter and her family.

These suffering experiences, the suffering condition, and the emotional responses of the frail elder are apprehended by others in Josephina's life-world—her roommate, the other residents, the care facility staff, her daughter. Suffering is intersubjectively experienced and is fundamentally social and relational in character. Consciousness of suffering is also consciousness of something other than suffering, an intentionality aimed at detaching oneself from suffering. In suffering there is an intentional movement away from suffering toward a transcendent state of being, a coming home to one's place of origin and connectedness to the Maternal dimensions of existence. Suffering threatens the horizon of experience and the possibility for transcendence. Josephina's testimony provides evidence of this intentional movement away from suffering in spiritual desires, intentionalities, and agentic processes to project a futural horizon for a relational self that transcends the existential condition.

Sense of spiritual well-being and self-care

In looking back on and reviewing her life, Josephina experiences a sense of spiritual well-being and self-fulfillment. She has had a "good life," a "happy life." This sense of well-being is related to expanded spatiality, going places, and enjoyment of the world:

> Well, that's all, that's it. I mean, I don't like the way I'm feeling. I would like to feel better. I wouldn't have the swelling. And I didn't get so tired. And besides, I get up at six o'clock in the morning. Six a.m. I'm in the dining area already. And then we eat about almost nine. And we have a nice breakfast. And we have bacon on Sunday. We have a very good breakfast; it's the best. And then the meals aren't too bad, but you get tired, they repeat. The same thing every such and such a day.
>
> Yes, right my real unhappiness is being in the wheelchair and the problem with the swelling.

Josephina has an overall sense that things are good enough at the care facility. She expresses interest in and a desire for friendship, and pleasure and enjoyment in the sociality of friendship. She also reaps satisfaction from the recreational activities in which she participates. These are all praxes that involve agentic processes. She says that the meals are good and sometimes the best, but her real source of anguish is her leg and the edema, and being wheelchair-bound. She has a desire to improve her health and to get better.

Josephina clearly experiences a very heavy burden as a result of her chronic illnesses and conditions. She has congestive heart failure and is in chronic, persistent discomfort and pain because of the edema in her legs. She is also in chronic discomfort because of the diuretics she is taking for the edema. While she expresses confidence in the care she is receiving at the care facility, she understands the complexity of her state of health, involving all her systems, and that she has a role to play as a decision maker.

Relationships with health care professionals and trust in health care system

Josephina trusts the health care system and her professional caregivers. This trust is maintained despite repeated assaults on its integrity. Her testimony suggests her difficulty in establishing trusting relationships with direct care staff and with the nursing staff. However, she has a trusting relationship with her psychologist and is very comfortable with her recreational therapist. She has a relationship with her nurse practitioner, who informs her about her medications and any changes in them.

Josephina seems to regard the relationship with her social worker as instrumental in nature: if there is a certain task that needs to be done, such as the burial arrangements that have to be addressed, her social worker is available. However, Josephina does not communicate a strong sense of a deep, trusting relationship with her social worker or that her social worker is the health professional whom she would seek if she had a special concern that she wanted to share or discuss. She says that she does not have much conversation with her social worker, but "only some complaints." Josephina's transactional perspective of the social work role conveys the social and relational dimensions of her experiences in the care facility and the nature of structural support provided by the social work role.

Health care decisions and the decision making process

Josephina's involvement in medication decisions is an area fraught with conflict. Her uncertainty and unhappiness about her medication regimen and how it affects her functioning come up several times with respect to pain control, bowel function, and fluid retention. Josephina seems hesitant to challenge the good care she believes she is receiving from the care facility and the professionals in the care facility. However, she also feels she is "trying her best," or, in other words, is being a good resident and doing everything she is supposed to be doing. Josephina is problematizing this area of health care decision making and reflecting that she is involved in an agentic process.

Conclusion

In my interviews with this group of frail elders, I was struck by the diverse communities that I heard them describing—from the highly integrated community of women who belonged to religious orders to various other types of communities found in the care facility itself. These communities included peer-to-peer elder communities, and community sub-groups that shared common interests or goals—such as the resident council, meal-time congregate groups, and members of spiritual or prayer communities. These descriptions of communities resonated with testimony about the pervasive social isolation of elders receiving chronic care in facility environments, signaling in many instances the absence or disintegration of community. It is clear, however, that community is protective for vulnerable elders living in facility environments, and that working toward building stronger communities will help to prevent and relieve pervasive suffering among frail elders.

In these accounts provided by elderly persons receiving chronic care, we are honoring their voices and their perspectives. I as the researcher make no judgments about their existential positings, or the quality of care they are receiving in the respective facilities. I am focused only on understanding the experiences of the elders themselves—in particular, their experiences of suffering and how they are constituted. The testimonies in this chapter from these three elderly women disclose things about suffering experience and its intentional structure that I found remarkable—from the revelation by Virginia that deep meaning in life does not bring relief from suffering, to Bernadette's knowing gaze about what meaning the loss of community had for her, and finally to Josephina, for whom no suffering of her own could exceed the suffering she experienced in communion with her daughter and her family who were living in a shelter and in a state of total depletion, dependency and helplessness. Josephina's unbounded Maternal generosity to her daughter, and her choosing to be a moral agent in light of the suffering of her daughter and family, disclose the moral significance of the world. In these narratives, we see unbounded suffering being met by the unbounded surplus of Maternal grace.

7 Seriously Ill Older Adults in Recovery
Maternal Environments

The narratives in the preceding chapters describe the experiences of frail elderly women in their encounters with suffering, chronic pain, and serious illness. In this chapter, I turn to the narrative of Peter, an older adult man—in the young-old age range—who struggled with advanced illness, complex wounds and chronic pain, as well as several other men who were chronically wounded. These seriously ill men—whose bodily wounds transcended the physical—turned to the inpatient or residential care facility for maternal care even in the face of multiple traumas.

The Narrative of Peter: Intolerable Pain, Extreme Suffering and Recovery

One older adult (whom I shall call "Peter") was admitted to a facility's inpatient chronic wound care program. Peter presented with medically complex wounds and chronic pain, as well as impaired skin integrity in the lower extremities and a history of substance abuse. In a life-historical interview, Peter disclosed that before coming to the care facility, he experienced extreme suffering following a serious injury to his leg, resulting leg ulcerations and multiple surgeries, excruciating pain from debridement procedures and dressing removals, and stigma, shame, and loss of self related to the intolerable odor from his necrotic skin. The unbearable suffering and distress in living through these experiences led to his desire to die. After having been admitted to the facility, Peter described his much higher level of comfort in the caring environment of the facility and his confidence in the medical management of his wounds, and reflected in his communications, tone, and calm demeanor a recovered sense of dignity as well as hope. In addition, medical record data showed that, over the course of his inpatient stay from date of admission to discharge, Peter's appetite increased to 110 percent, pain levels decreased, and lower extremity wounds got smaller. In the four problem areas identified in Peter's care plan at admission—pain, impaired skin integrity, nutrition, and safety—improvements were documented in the period after admission. Peter is one of several elders in these narratives who turns to the care facility for the Maternal care he has not found in the world outside the institution. This is a reversal of the way things are ordinarily expected to go, but not entirely uncommon, and increasingly becoming more common among seriously ill, vulnerable persons who have limited resources and are relieved to find a home, a room of their own, a clean bed and sheets, and nourishing food in a facility that most would want to avoid.

The dignity-affirming care that was part of Peter's palliative management in the care facility to which he was admitted included attention and attunement to his bodily, emotional and spiritual needs, monitoring his reports of pain and pain relief after adjustments to pain medications, careful cleaning and dressing of his wounds to prevent pain and eliminate odor, and creation of a space in which he was able to feel honored and valued by those bearing witness to his pain and suffering. These findings demonstrate the impact of relational, dignity-affirming care on health outcomes in one population of seriously ill older adults. This particular individual was a member of a subgroup of elders with advanced illness and complex wounds.

Peter's experience in the care facility varied from the seriously ill elderly women in these chapter narratives in that *he turned to the facility* for the care that he had not been able to secure on the outside. As a result, he did not experience the same level of traumatic dislocation in the transfer to the facility in the way Angelique, Camila, Jospehina and many of the elderly women did. There were other aspects of Peter's experience that were traumatic for him and caused him distress, but the institutional environment was not chief among them. Rather, Peter flourished as a result of the care he received in the facility environment. Had he not been transferred to the facility, he would probably have suffered a premature death, as he himself acknowledged. Peter's transfer to the facility rescued him from abject poverty and other social conditions that jeopardized his safety, health and well-being. Peter's situation was not dissimilar to the circumstances of Harvey, a male resident also in the young-old age range, who had suffered a partial leg amputation and experienced relief in coming to a care facility not only to receive medical care, but also to be fed, bathed, and housed in a warm, clean room of his own. Both Peter and Harvey are examples of individuals who experienced accelerated aging as a result of their chronic illness burden and exposure to life-course traumas.

I would return to visit Peter several times over the course of three months to conduct the interviews that were a part of my research study. Each interview was lengthy. On the occasions when I visited him and he was unable to participate in actual interviews, we would still spend a few minutes chatting. He was always delighted to receive the visits and to have the opportunity to update me on what was happening with his situation.

Descriptions of Suffering and Chronic Pain

I first met Peter in the fall of the year, shortly after he was admitted to the facility. Before we had any conversation, I was struck upon first entering room by the seriousness of his illness. He was in bed, his head only slightly inclined, and his feet protruded from the covers at the end of the bed, wrapped in white dressing cloths. Although he seemed like a tall man, he was gaunt and emaciated-looking, with hollows in his cheeks. Despite his ill condition, he was very welcoming, invited me to sit, and easily engaged in conversation with me about my study for the purposes of the informed consent process. He was eager to participate in the study. As we began to go through and complete the informed consent process, Peter had already begun to tell his story.

Peter's medical needs involved complex care because of an advanced illness process and necrotic skin from ulcerations on his lower extremities that caused him unbearable pain at times. Although his extremities were wrapped, he freely offered pictures of his wounds so that I would fully appreciate the extent of his suffering. He described a deteriorating medical situation that was accompanied by a sense of hopelessness and despair prior to his admission to the inpatient chronic wound program, where he was now being treated and receiving chronic care:

> This is me in the hospital [acute care hospital]. They had me sedated and I was saying, "Man, I don't want no more of that Demerol and all that stuff." You can see how I had had it. This is how my legs looked before he did the debriding. All this is dead skin. [I was in] a lot of discomfort. Yeah, and see how big it is. This one here is the worst. This is the one right here where it's all right down on my foot and up my leg. [Showing pictures to researcher.] Oh, and see all that dead—and it stunk. Oh, it stunk.
>
> Oh, bad odor. See, all this you could see here... and all that blackness is where it was dead skin and they had to get it out, you know, because when I was home, my wife would help me change my bandages and I would change them, and like within three hours the odor was back, you know, and it made me sick. I was throwing up. I couldn't get adjusted to that odor, man. I mean, it was so horrific. Then, the flies started getting attracted to my leg, you know. Both of us are saying, "Where are they coming from?" We had all the windows closed but, you know, them flies are wonders when they want to get to something dead because—then I wind up getting maggots in it.
>
> One night, I said, "Oh, what's that on my foot?" So, I was screaming, man, and calling my wife and we tore the bandages off and she screamed and backed up because it took her a while to get adjusted to doing my legs because, you know, you see how they looking. She was with me when my legs wasn't like that. So, when she seen the maggots on my leg, it was horrific for both of us. I was depressed. I started crying. I said, "Why is this happening to me?"
>
> They had this thing they call solution, bleach solution. And you spray it on the leg and boy, I mean, it burns. Oh, God, it burns and I get howling, you know, and trying to wait for it to stop. It goes for like five or seven minutes of that intense burning and I'd be howling, wiping my face, sweating. I mean, it was horrible, but it killed the maggots. We went right to the doctor, Dr. X, the next day. He said, "Peter, you have to have the surgery to debride this because you're going to lose your leg." Now, he ain't heard nothing from Dr. Z. This was his conclusion.
>
> They took the bullet out, the fragments and Dr. X said, "Peter, you're going to lose your legs, man, if you don't listen to me and do what I tell you

to do." He said, "I can't cut no corners with you. The signs are there. You got large areas of dead tissue, and the dead tissue is not just yellow, it's black. So now it's telling me that it's going to infect your bone in the areas where it's black at." You can see how many areas I had on there that was black. He said, "Then you had the maggots on there. You have to go and have surgery immediately. You can't wait. You've got to do this right away."

So, I said, "All right, Dr. X." We set up an appointment. I don't have no choice. Then, I wind up falling at the restaurant.

Peter gave very graphic descriptions of the chronic and unbearable pain he suffered through these ordeals, and how his pain affected his emotional, mental and spiritual health:

I didn't want to live no more. I didn't want to live no more. I was like at that point. My wife heard me one time in there crying. She was in the bathroom. I didn't know she was up there. I thought she was in the kitchen. I said, "I can't take this no more. I can't. I don't want to live like this. My body is falling apart." Everything was depressing and I couldn't eat. The pain was so intense.

Yes. I mean, [the pain was] beyond unbearable. It would break me up at night. I would have muscle spasms and it would squeeze my legs and I would just be shaking and sweating and going through all those different degrees of depression. It was making me feel like I don't want to be on this earth anymore. It was very difficult.

Peter's descriptions of living with the odor of his dead skin is a compelling account of pain in all its dimensions—alienating Peter from his own lived body and heightening his suffering to a level that he finds so unbearable that he vomits:

He [Dr. X.] said, "Peter, we can't do this no more. You have to go to surgery, because I'm just inflicting unnecessary pain on you. You don't deserve that." So, I said, "I totally agree with you, Dr. X. I don't want to go through this," but he got enough off to where it toned down the smell and it didn't smell for a few days until it came back.

Oh, like dead dogs or dead rats, horrible. I mean, I threw up numerous times, it got me so sick. I mean, I used to have a wash cloth over my nose to stay away from all that smell because it was so intense. Sometimes I would be laying back while my wife was doing it. I come up and I see that. There'd be tears in her eyes and stuff. She's saying, "My love, what's wrong? I don't want to see you go through no more pain. It's been too long."

These accounts of the complex dialectics and feedback mechanisms of chronic pain at work, for Peter, go beyond biological tissue damage in fully implicating his emotional, psychological, social, cultural, and spiritual systems. Peter's total pain experience, which in its multidimensionality is intentionally directed toward his own lived body and his field of embodied pain, heaps more unrelenting pain on him, alienating him from the very body and the only body through which he may engage with the world. Peter experiences a loss of corporeality. This total pain experience is also not a totally passive experience for Peter, but one in which he becomes actively engaged with his whole intentional being.

We also see in Peter's accounts and descriptions that, prior to coming to the care facility, he is living in chronic pain. There is no abatement of his pain, and no interventions are able to bring him relief from it. This situation of chronic pain is one of clear and certain suffering for Peter. He does not need to tell his loved ones or caregivers "I am suffering," although he does that through many different forms of communication. But he need not rely on language alone to communicate the depths of his suffering because it is palpable and undeniable. We see it and apprehend it in all of its terrible and unspeakable reality. Although we can never occupy Peter's own temporal stream of consciousness, our intuitive seeing and passive synthesis and assimilation of his experience is more than enough for us to empathically access and inform our understanding of his suffering.

In the movement from pain that can be controlled and managed to unbearable pain and unrelieved suffering, there is also a loss of passivity for the suffering person. Embodied pain and suffering, which are always lived through in the lived body and the body's field of experience, turn the suffering elder toward the lived body and the self in a way that is brutally reflexive—hyper-reflexivity that takes the elder person out of the mode of pre-reflective, passive assimilation in the common sense world. A leg that is necrotic is no longer a leg as we understand it in our common sense knowledge. It is a leg that has become the center of the person's life-world, so much so that the person can no longer tolerate its very presence, nor tolerate his own embodied self. This preoccupation with self—and sometimes preservation of self—are is also a form of non-availability, or in Marcel's (1949) words, "non-disposability" (p. 69).

In this stage of Peter's illness, we see one example of the pathway from pain to suffering. Pain and suffering are co-present, and intolerable and intractable pain leads to more intense pain and unrelieved suffering. Unrelieved pain and suffering involve annihilation for the suffering elder—for Peter, annihilation of self and his intentional connection with the world. This pathway is one of many pathways to suffering. The second phase of Peter's illness trajectory, during which time he received chronic care in the facility, brings variation in his experience.

Descriptions of Healing and Recovery: Turning to Facility for Maternal Care

By early winter, when I visited Peter, there had been a major change in his illness course. He described the positive direction of his healing process:

> Well, I'm doing a lot better. Yeah, I'm gaining weight. I've been eating everything. My appetite is back.
>
> [The healing process], it's going real good. I had—they've been giving me this protein. Yeah. And I've been drinking that. Yeah. Everybody says they

don't understand how I can do that because they usually put it in milk or food. Even the doctor said how you can drink that straight. To me, it don't bother me. It's been helping me heal. It's been helping me heal.

So, I brought up my walker because I'm ready to get out of this bed and start walking. No, [I have not gotten up yet]. But I've been exercising. Therapist has been here. They started the therapy. And the days she don't come, I still do the therapy. And she was doing like these here—10 this way, 10 this way. I'm doing 50 now. She said, "Wow, you really stepped it up." I said, "Yeah."

I feel better.

I observed Peter's marked improvements, not only in his presenting physical appearance, weight gain, and more erect posture in his bed, but in his attitude of confidence and optimism about the course of his recovery. I also observed his feet protruding in the same way from under the covers as they had when I first encountered him, but now I could see that his toes had fresh skin on them. There was no evidence of the hopelessness and despair that I had sensed when I first interviewed him in early November. He was no longer in a state of chronic pain and unbearable suffering from his complex wounds. The facility staff were effectively managing his pain—which was now more episodic—based on Peter's self-reports.

Here we see that Peter was still struggling with pain at times, but it was no longer the type of pain that became intolerable and intractable, and would lead to the unbearable suffering he had experienced before. His pain was being managed and controlled.

However, even though Peter did not manifest or describe unbearable pain and suffering, there were aspects of his conversations with me that suggested that he continued to experience forms of suffering that were not related in any way to the pain associated with tissue damage. The suffering he experienced centered around his life-situation, his relations with his wife, and concerns about her welfare. For example, he experienced high levels of distress both when he learned that his wife had to be admitted to a hospital for open heart surgery not long after he had been admitted to the chronic care facility, and throughout her post-surgical recovery period. When I saw him last, he expressed significant distress about his house having been robbed and the sense of violation that accompanied this event. These experiences of psychological and emotional distress are forms of suffering, and may themselves cause somatic symptoms or pain. A third example of distress that Peter described was associated with being bedridden after many months in hospitals, and not yet being able to walk. He reflected upon the time he had spent in his earlier life biking alongside his wife during her runs, and he yearned for the freedom to pursue these activities again.

Michael was also a seriously ill elder with complex wounds admitted to the inpatient chronic wound care program facility. He had been transferred from an acute care hospital after being told by one of his doctors that it was time, "to cut off his leg." Michael refused such proposed treatment. Like Peter, he was also bedbound, struggling with advanced illness processes, and was waiting for his legs to heal. The new team at the facility to which he was transferred gave him hope that he was indeed healing.

Even though Michael and Peter shared a somewhat similar medical history, with complex wounds and diagnoses of chronic disease, their experiences of pain and suffering varied. Michael did not report being in chronic pain. Rather, most of the time his pain was short and episodic, and had the quality of boundedness. He would even go so far as to say that he had no pain, only discomfort:

> I don't have pain. I don't have pain.
>
> Yeah, discomfort, being restricted to this bed. This is going to be the first year that I haven't been around family for Christmas, since I was born. Even when I went away to school and stuff, seeing everybody, all sides of the family at this time of year is always very important.
>
> Yeah, the first year. I mean, my wife has been very, very good. I give her a lot of credit. She tries to get up here at least once a week, maybe twice a week. She's been very good about it. She can't drive at night anymore, so she comes up in the daytime.
>
> Christmas, I don't know about. Maybe my wife, but—what's today? Today is Friday. Sunday, my side of the family is going to have a get-together. They're coming from Massachusetts and Jersey and upstate New York. It's my brothers and sisters and nephews. They're going to meet by my brother's house. He rented the hall in the basement of his building. They'll bring— everybody will bring something and then, they'll have it partially catered.
>
> [I am] a little down in the dumps.

Michael did reluctantly acknowledge some pain:

> When I first came in, if they touched my left foot, it was very, very painful. I had three operations on the feet, and the skin was—you touched it, I jumped. So, I took painkillers when I first came in. Now, when they change the dressing, I don't take any pain pills.
>
> Yes. But I did have two days where I had like a—what's the best way to... [a stabbing pain], right above the toes, the middle toes on the right foot. But then, all of a sudden, it disappeared and I didn't—so I took painkillers for two days and that has been all that I've taken in all the time I've been here.
>
> Two days and then, it went away.
>
> Well, [before coming to the facility] the left foot was sore.
>
> Three different operations. The left foot had three. I don't remember if the right foot had three or just two... Only when they went to—the last time, I believe they actually took some bone out of the left foot. It was very, very sensitive to any—my foot was—every time anybody touched me. It was very sensitive. But it seems to be fine now. They can change the dressing and work on it down there and it doesn't bother me.

These accounts convey that Michael's pain, when he experienced it, was resolved. It did not develop into a full-blown chronic condition. However, what was not resolved is what he called discomfort. This discomfort, which was not directly related to any tissue damage, was a form of distress and suffering and qualitatively different than his episodic pain because the discomfort was unbounded, contextual. Michael explained that his discomfort was related primarily to his being confined to bed. This was his suffering, and it was not relieved because he did not know when his confinement to bed would end or when he would be restored to being a fully whole human being.

Even in light of this suffering that Michael described while in the care facility, he also spoke of many of the same things that Peter found nourishing in the facility environment:

> We had a nice luncheon the other day, on Wednesday. What did they call it? Noel. And the food was—I didn't even eat the main course. I filled up on the appetizers.
>
> Yeah. And the band they had was, the band donates their time, and they had a singer come in that was different from the band, dressed a little bit like Elvis Presley, and he was good. And then after that the police marching band came in, the bagpipers.
>
> To a point. They can blow you out. My brother is in a bagpipe band, electrical union. So these guys were a little better than his. In fact, they had at least 16 bagpipers, and six or eight drummers.
>
> [It was in] the room downstairs, the big room, but even down there it was loud.
>
> Yeah. My wife was here.
>
> Yeah. [I got into] a wheelchair—they had trouble getting me in that last week. They almost killed my right leg. They didn't hold it and it started to bend, and then I couldn't get it right. Then I got cramps up here.
>
> Yeah, we went down there. We stayed down until I told my wife, I've got to go back upstairs. I think I'm going to have to go to the bathroom soon. There's no way downstairs I can get up.
>
> Yeah, they did a nice job, the volunteers and everybody else.

While Michael suffered losses of family, community and social life in coming to the facility, and experienced a traumatic dislocation as a result, once he became acclimated to the facility, he, like Peter, turned to the new environment as a source of nourishment.

Building a Hospitable Cosmos

My encounter with Barney is unforgettable. I was told that he was an elderly gentleman with complex, chronic wounds, and was interested in speaking with me about participating in the study. I had no inkling at that time that his interests in speaking would go well beyond the purposes of the study. When I first met him and introduced myself, he was most welcoming. I felt at home with him immediately. But the informed consent process was the most labor-intensive I had yet experienced with any potential study participant. Barney was clearly in a great deal of discomfort and craved the engagement and social intercourse that was part of the interview process. He asked me to read the informed consent out loud to him line by line. Slowly, we worked our way through it—I responding to his questions about various possible scenarios, in particular concerning confidentiality. He also wanted to see the scale measures we would be working with. I could see he was pleased that I was willing to take time to answer all his questions as fully as possible. At one point, a staff person entered the room while we were doing the informed consent, and he became quite agitated. After the staff person left, he shared that her presence in the room heightened his anxiety and distress. He expressed fear that in her brusqueness and insensitivity, he might be exposed to harm in his already very vulnerable condition. After about an hour and a half, he was so tired that we couldn't complete the informed process that day. I left the informed consent and scale measures with him to review further and assured him I would visit again to continue our conversation.

It was a couple of weeks before I was able to return, and when I did it took some time before Barney remembered who I was. On this second visit, he was sitting in a chair and was drinking his protein drink, but insisted I proceed with the interview conversation. We went through the same rituals as before, with his seeking my assistance in positioning his computer in a certain place, as well as his meal tray, and various items on the tray. As taxing and anxiety-provoking as these rituals were for me because of my dread apprehension I would, without intention, do something to cause him distress, I was deeply empathic with the desperateness of his situation. After he signed the informed consent, he described the discomfort he had in his shoulders, his swollen belly, and his ulcerated legs and feet. He also spoke about losing his wife, who had died of cancer in the very facility where he was now receiving care. Barney turned to me several times during his story and asked me, seemingly in jest but with pathos-filled eyes, "Are you crying yet?"

It became clear in a relatively short time, though, that Barney had things he wanted to tell me—how he got there, the ordeals he had been through with surgery and post-surgical renal failure. But he was most interested in talking about the care environment, and he wanted to know if this was an area that I wanted to explore. I let him guide our conversation, and he explained to me how his experience of the care he received influenced his experience of comfort or discomfort, relief or heightened distress. He shared his observations that the staff who came into contact with his body were not as highly trained as the doctors who came to see him and never touched him. He described how his skin was ripped off sometimes during the dressing changes when the staff did not take enough care with this procedure. He said that there were many staff who provided good care and whom he was happy to see when they entered the room Even though Barney indicated that he had heightened anxiety when certain staff entered his room, he communicated through his bodily presence in the room that he had made the facility his home. He relished not only his meal encounters, but encounters with staff he trusted. And he exhibited no reluctance in voicing his needs and how he wanted them met. He actively engaged with his environment and worked to cultivate it as a "hospitable threshold" (Jager, 1999, p. 19)—from use of equipment, such as his computer and urinal, to inhabiting a cosmos with his wife who died in the facility and was spiritually present to him."

In the midst of our conversation, he indicated that he needed to use the urinal. He asked me to locate it on the bed and give it to him, which I did. I left the room quickly so he could relieve himself. When I returned, he asked me to take the urinal and place it on a table. He seemed embarrassed, but I assured him the presence of the urine did not trouble me.

I asked Barney about his pain. He said he did not know if he was receiving any pain medications. He said his children probably knew. This led him to describe his doctor's patterns of communication with his son, who was his health care agent. He felt he was not made a part of these conversations about his goals of care. The doctor would speak with his son before he spoke to him. Barney would continue to build his cosmos in the facility, and negotiate the roles of host and guest in his new environment and in meeting the challenges of communication between patient and caregivers, as well as the many others that he would undoubtedly face.

Transcending Conditions of Human Finitiude

In one of my last visits to the facility site, I was encouraged by the staff to introduce myself to Chris. The door to Chris's room was closed, so I hesitated to disturb him. When I knocked on the door and heard his voice inviting me in, I entered with some trepidation. I found a handsome, younger looking man (in the young-old age range) sitting up in his bed, and a family member sitting by the window. Chris was very welcoming, insisted on my sitting down, and expressed immediate interest in speaking with me. We worked through the informed consent process painlessly and moved quickly into conversation. Chris was entirely open about his illness experiences, and as he spoke, I was uplifted by his spirit—cheerful and pleasant, engaging with staff when they came into the room, and chatting brightly about his pottery projects that adorned the room. The room emitted a brightness too: the wall behind his head was painted yellow, but I am sure much of this aura of light came from Chris himself.

This light stood in stark contrast to the "unspeakable"—yes, "unspeakable" assaults Chris had suffered to his lived body. He told me the story of being an iron worker and some time ago having experienced discomfort in his back, which he at first attributed to the type of work he did. The early diagnosis was a herniated disk. After going for a number of medical tests and evaluations, he received the dire news that he had sarcoma, a type of cancer. The cancer had invaded his body in a way that made it not easily accessible to surgical procedures. However, he did go through a 14-hour surgery after refusing a leg amputation, and after about 13 years the cancer returned. Radiation treatment resulted in damage to his bones and skin, infection, and an open wound in his back that led to his transfer to the care facility where he was residing when I encountered him. He described terrible pain, but indicated that it was being controlled with both oral and IV medications now that he was an inpatient. He showed me the tumor that was growing on his side, which he described as a small basketball. The tumor was as large as he had said, taped and hidden from view, but nevertheless attached to his body and holding him hostage. He reported that it interfered with his mobility.

Chris also spoke about his family. His wife was with him by his bedside, devotedly, and was living round the clock in the room with him. He spoke of his two adopted children who came to see him often, one of whom was still at home, and of visits with his granddaughter who brought him great joy. I sensed that it was a challenge of enormous proportions to maintain a home from a distance while living full-time in a facility. However, none of these challenges seemed to dampen Chris's optimism and hope. I observed in his interactions with the staff that they were as visibly affected by Chris as I was, totally engaged and caring in their responsiveness to him. It was clear that even in the face of unspeakable bodily wounds, Chris transcended his conditions of human finitude.

Chris wore a heavy gold cross around his neck and bare chest. I asked him if this cross had a special meaning for him. He shared with me that it was a gift from his mother and father, and that his mother had passed away recently also from cancer. This was the only moment I was with him that I sensed a deep sadness. I departed Chris with a very heavy heart, and hoped that I would have the pleasure of spending more time with him in a future visit. I understood that in Chris's presence, even as researcher, I was a witness to much more than my pain and suffering—I participated during the moment of my encounter with Chris in his spiritual transcendence.

Conclusion

All four of the men whose narrative accounts are shared in this chapter lived through the traumatic experience, among others, of being told by a physician that they would need to have a leg amputated or "cut off," and each one of them refused the leg amputation as a proposed treatment option. These refusals—not only to accept treatment, but also refusal to accept the authority of the medical establishment—were examples of brave agentic action and decision making that revealed the presence of an autonomous self. Peter and Michael made near miraculous recoveries in the caring environment of the care facility with aggressive wound care and pain management. Their wounds healed enough to permit them to be discharged to a lower level of care. By recovery, I mean not only the partial healing of physical wounds which were previously evaluated as leaving no option but amputation, but also recovery of an emotional, social and spiritual character as well. Barney's and Chris's illness trajectories continued to be a source of suffering for them, but they struggled to cultivate types of well-being. While the individual experiences of pain and suffering among all four older men varied, there were central aspects of their suffering experiences—even for Chris, the youngest of this group of participants—that emerged as prominent and essential to suffering, namely, losses of dignity-affirming care and Maternal Foundations in profound suffering that led to their empathic care-seeking drive for healing, resilience and recovery.

Among all of the study-participants discussed in these narratives, Chris and Harvey, who were selected as comparison cases, were the youngest among the older adult study participants. One of the ways Harvey's experience differed from the other four persons discussed in this chapter, however, is that he did suffer the partial loss of a leg. While his experience of suffering fit within the general structure in which Maternal dimensions of existence were prominent, like Peter, Harvey turned to the facility environment as a source of Maternal care, comfort and soothing, and to replace the empathic care and security he had not found outside the nursing home. He was the only person I interviewed in the study who exhibited a different type of intentional striving toward well-being within the same general structure of suffering. Phenomenologically, I saw vividly with Harvey the lived, expressive, and weeping body, his palpable and visible bodily pain and suffering as he lay in his bed in the facility—his amputated limb, his ulcerated heel, and his writhing body that ached to be free of the burden of illness. But unlike Peter, Michael, Barney and Chris, Harvey demonstrated much more of a collapsed agency in the face of his existential suffering and was unable to mobilize his personal resources to recover from his losses or accommodate changes in his life-world. He persisted in refusing to get out of bed and remained steadfast in his desire to stay in the confines of his room. Harvey stood out among all the persons I interviewed as perhaps the only individual who appeared to desire death—death as a type of well-being—even in the midst of the good care he received in the care facility.

My last visits to the facility sites, Peter and Michael were no longer inpatients. They had been discharged to lower levels of care. The palliative treatments they had received as inpatients not only relieved their pain, but were healing for them. Barney remained in the facility. The wound care he was receiving was palliative in controlling his pain and managing his complex wounds. I was not as optimistic that Barney would have the same miraculous healing that Peter and Michael experienced with their chronic wounds. But a chaplain stopped in to see him when I was with him, and he invited her to come back to speak with him the next day. His healing would perhaps be spiritual, if not physical, as he continued to receive good symptom management.

8 Conclusion

A Call for Broader Social Care Provision – A Maternal Turn in Ethics of Care

The foregoing narratives in this book provide compelling accounts of suffering experience—women and men from diverse backgrounds and cultures, as they live through chronic, serious illness and chronic pain. These accounts have important implications for individuals who face serious physical or mental illness, and for the development and articulation of public policy—as well as for future directions in public health research, practice, and bioethical inquiry and its applications in the field. From negotiating conflicts at the bedside to the design of more humanistic, Maternal care environments, sensitivity to pain and suffering experiences must inform, and be informed by, human understanding across disciplines and sectors.

Both first-person and more global, social ecological perspectives allow the voices of seriously ill persons in the suffering narratives to speak for themselves through the lens of phenomenology, drawing on the phenomenological tradition in Husserl, as well as Schutz, Merleau-Ponty, Levinas and others who followed him. It is the goal of phenomenology in this project to open up a space for empathically accessing and recovering the unheralded and invisible social worlds of suffering as they are revealed in the lived experiences of women and men in aging and serious illness. Drawing attention to, and making visible and explicit, the unthematized, everyday social practices, habits and meanings of persons who are suffering helps to guide and shape policy, improve the design of care systems, and prevent and relieve suffering.

Over the last three decades, professionals across many disciplines—policy, law, research, public health, social work, psychology, medicine, nursing, chaplaincy, and ethics—have begun to concern themselves with issues of pain, suffering, and dislocation among seriously ill and frail elders, their family caregivers, and the communities in which they are situated. Older adults are affected by diverse forms of trauma, loss, grief or social suffering, such as may be inflicted by disasters. Only incremental progress has been made, however, in understanding experiences of chronic pain and suffering, identifying and meeting person- and family-centered goals of care, and relieving pain and suffering—in part through the advancement and growth of palliative care as a philosophy and a discipline, and through promotion of community resilience perspectives. Myriad significant barriers remain to the adequate assessment, treatment and understanding of pain and suffering due to social structural factors and gaps in policy and research (Institute of Medicine, 2011), perhaps chief among them the concomitant failures to explicitly recognize pain and suffering as issues that affect the the the public's health, and to fashion appropriate, therapeutic policy responses to address them in their full magnitude. Even independent of these policy failures, the complexity of human suffering continues to remain a vastly unexamined, uncharted, and understudied universe of lived experience in its full biopsychosocial and ethical dimensions, in particular, with respect to the nature of our ethical obligation as human beings and as a society to those who suffer.

The chapter narratives are not case studies, but examples of suffering that share the same general structure, and also identify mid-level generality or types of experiences, such as experiences of care facilities as Maternal environments. The constituents of the general structure, as presented in the narrative accounts, integrate the findings into a reframed understanding of human suffering. In so doing, the findings may contribute to current knowledge, and place this knowledge in the larger context of provision and ethics of care in this twenty-first century. The tentative suggestions about the findings revealed in the narratives may invite engagement and dialogue by members of diverse communities, including scholars, scientists, and health professionals and caregivers.

General Structure of Suffering in the Narrative Accounts

Suffering among seriously ill elderly women and men living in care facilities is a multifaceted experience—personal, intersubjective, and social developmental— that involves many contexts, social systems, and environments. The Maternal Ground, and the systems of agency, sociality and spirituality that form foundations that rest on the Maternal, are the constituents or blocks of granite that undergird the fabric and texture of suffering. Agency, in its variegated forms, may be a palliative response to suffering that permits seriously ill elderly persons to recover lost Maternal Foundations and their constitutive empathy, comfort, and security, as well as to attain varying levels of self-acceptance, accommodation to change, and resilience while living with serious and life-limiting illness. Immature personal development, weakened perceptions of self-efficacy due to past experiences with failure, and spiritual alienation may interfere with agentic drives for self-actualization at the end of life. The suffering of seriously ill elderly women and men and their agentic responses to illness burden as they near the end of life surpass the limitations of illness and ultimately concern the tasks, hopes and challenges of taking on the mantle of freedom as autonomous moral agents in a social world.

There are three temporal moments of suffering identified in the suffering narratives in both the individual and general structures of elders' suffering experiences: a temporal moment of a Maternal Ground which founds human development; a central moment of pain and suffering in which losses of Maternal Foundations and agency are invariant; and a third temporal moment in which persons strive for recovery of agency, spiritual well-being and a Maternal homecoming at the end of life even while living through suffering. Within this temporal structure of suffering, the founding, genetic constitution and temporalizing of suffering are critical to understanding suffering experience. The founding order in the structure of suffering, going back to its beginnings in a Maternal Ground, has significance because it speaks to the social developmental contexts of suffering that heretofore have not been adequately explored. The Maternal Ground is a first moment in experience that constitutes suffering in the experiences of these elderly persons and without which suffering would not occur or the experiences of suffering would collapse. Each constituent that makes up the general structure of suffering experience is defined conceptually as a self-contained but fluid system—a finite province of meaning—in open exchange with surrounding systems and the environment. This structure is consistent with social ecological theory and ecophenomenology that both take account of all forms of development in the cultural world (Embree, 2003), dynamic change across diverse systems, and knowledge about human development across the lifespan. The narratives reveal that chronically ill elderly persons may experience various types of resilience, recovery of agency, and possibility for change (Greene & Cohen, 2005; Nelson-Becker, 2006) and development—even when faced with declining states of health and functioning and in their very last days.

The chapter narratives expand the existing knowledge of suffering in revealing that suffering has a complex, social developmental structure. A deepening understanding of lived experiences of suffering among elderly women and men, exploring possibilities for human development in these experiences from the perspectives of seriously ill and frail elderly themselves, invites investigation of experiences and meanings of pain and their relationship to suffering and end-of-life decision making. The studies placed these experiences and care needs of seriously ill older adults in their life-historical contexts.

The theoretical and conceptual frameworks for the narratives drew upon the work of Bronfenbrenner (1979) and others who followed him and built on social ecological systems theory and its relationship to human development, including Carol Meyer (1983), who was responsible for establishing the critical importance of the ecosystems perspective to social work practice. The premise of the theoretical and conceptual frameworks, bracketed during data collection and analysis but used in helping to understand the findings, is that meaning-making in the life-worlds of seriously, ill elderly persons occurs in a social context, not in isolation. An elderly woman or man forms an identity as a suffering person (Morrissey, 2011a) and may make decisions in interacting with relational others, family caregivers, and social work and other health care professionals who are members of an interdisciplinary team. The interpretation of findings also drew upon the work of Emmanuel Levinas (1969, 1981) and his elaboration of interpersonal ethics, as well as Edmund Husserl (1970, 1989) and those who followed him. Levinas's approach stands in stark contrast to the political economy perspective that positions older adults as objects of commodification, privatization and medicalization processes in a bureaucratized medical industrial complex (Estes, 2001). The focus of the research studies that informed the narratives was the social and relational dimensions of lived experiences of suffering of elderly women and men.

The primary contribution of these narratives is in helping to elaborate the structure of suffering among chronically, seriously ill elderly women and men in care facilities and contributing to the body of knowledge. While the focus of phenomenology, phenomenological reflection and the methodological tools that are utilized in service of reflection and accessing human consciousness are theoretical, the knowledge that is gained through these research studies may help to inform the work of health care practitioners and family caregivers in practical spheres. The suffering of seriously ill persons with life-limiting and life-threatening illness are pressing concerns for health care practitioners and family caregivers. Seriously ill elderly women and men are faced with making difficult decisions about their care choices at the end of life that are complex and pose significant challenges for policy, practice, and research. Those choices involve not just the range of health care decisions that relate to care planning, goals of care, and evaluation of treatment options, but the moral experience and moral life of very sick and frail elders that underlie these more visible choices: the relationship and responsibility to the other, even in states of disability and compromise, and the trust placed in the other from whom the frail elder seeks empathic, Maternal care.

The social, health, and demographic characteristics of these populations of elderly women and men living in care facilities are such that their needs demand special attention. As a stronger evidence base has developed documenting the multimorbidity and frailty of elderly persons, the urgency and scope of the social and public health problem presented by their suffering experiences calls for an informed scientific and ethical response. Decision making for the seriously ill elderly involves individual, interpersonal, family, social, and ethical considerations, as well as interactions between and among various ecological systems. Social workers, psychologists, nurses, and other health practitioners are turning to palliative care as a well-recognized interdisciplinary approach that makes contributions to better practices in shared decision making (Bomba, Morrissey, & Leven, 2011), and helps to relieve suffering consistent with person-centered values and ethical principles (Blacker & Christ, 2011; Higgins, 2011).

Suffering among seriously ill elderly women and men demonstrates the dimensions of the phenomena from the perspectives of the seriously ill elderly themselves currently situated in care facilities and in multiple social roles, as persons involved in decision making, members of a community, and as family members: daughters, mothers, fathers, brothers, sisters, aunts, grandmothers, great-grandmothers. In-depth interviews with elderly persons reveal the challenges posed by living with serious, chronic illness in highly complex, structured institutional environments. Two types of experience emerge in the narratives among elderly persons within the general structure of suffering: the experience of the care facility as Maternal, and the experience of the transition from home to institution as traumatic. For some, both of these experiences may be present at once to the extent there are certain aspects of the care facility environment that are Maternal, and others that may give rise to losses of Maternal Foundations.

All of the elderly persons in the suffering narratives found comfort and soothing in the Maternal dimensions of existence and sought Maternal empathic care in multiple domains. Angelique and Peter found comfort in the food they ate. Food had a specific meaning for them that was Maternal in nature, providing nurturance, welcome, soothing, and security. Angelique asked the care facility staff to make her tea and in her tea she finds solace. Peter, Harvey, and Alejandro derived comfort from the food, and experienced the care facility itself to be a homelike environment and source of Maternal care. Ann and Peggy found Maternal comfort in cigarette smoking, providing regular and constant support for them even when they experienced other types of distress.

Camila's and Josephina's life-histories revealed subtly different individual structures of suffering at the end of their lives. Camila, an elderly Latina woman, revealed a higher level of well-being than her peers in the care facility. It is not entirely clear whether this pattern of well-being was related to her more robust health, her not being wheelchair- or bed-bound, or to other factors influencing her well-being—such as a stronger sense of spiritual meaning, strong perceptions of self-efficacy, the quality of her social relationships, or cultural factors. Many elders demonstrated that they were able to hold feelings of well-being at the same time that they experienced suffering. These feelings of well-being that were rooted in, and brought the Maternal dimensions of existence to bear, sustained these frail elders in their suffering.

Josephina had a powerful sense of agency and self-efficacy related to her daughter and her family and how she desired to provide support to them. She maintained regular contact with them by phone. Tawanda experienced satisfaction in being able to perform self-care functions and not having to be dependent on the care facility staff, as well as being able to help her roommate. Camila, Josephina, Tawanda, Ann and Ruth described "going places," both within the four walls and sometimes outside the care facility, making excursions to shopping malls and ball games—Ann's "going to the garden" every day to seek the company of her friends, and Ruth's "going places" even from her bed as she watched the TV and imagined her journeys.

Discussion of General Structure of Suffering of Seriously Ill Older Women and Men

The structure of suffering is generalized to seriously ill elderly women and men who have chronic, serious illness or are approaching the end of life, and living in care facilities. The suffering narratives also have relevance to elderly persons living in the community and to non-elderly persons with serious illness or serious mental illness, subject to the methodological limitations explained in Chapter 1. The invariant feature of the general structure is the Maternal Ground.

First Temporal Moment: Maternal Ground

The meaning of the Maternal Ground for seriously ill frail and non-frail elderly women and men approaching the end of life has complexity. LaCoursiere (2010) reported findings from a small qualitative study of hospice workers indicating that

10–25 percent of deaths provided evidence of dying callings to "mother." These studies expand upon these findings in demonstrating that persons' experiences of suffering at the end of life are founded upon a Maternal Ground in which they invoke the security and comfort of the Maternal at the end of life. Elders revealed their retentions and re-enactments of Maternal experiences. Recollections of these experiences by elders helped them to recreate the Maternal Ground in the care facility to cope with their suffering experiences and soothe their pain. Essential manifestations or instantiations of the Maternal Ground from which other systems of experience in the lives of suffering persons spring forth are empathy, receptivity, relational intimacy and generosity, unconditional loving care, a welcoming home that is protective, palliative and assures well-being, desire, and generativity.

The Maternal is a pervasive experience and a frame of reference for elders as the origin of social development (Geniusas, 2010). Elders recollect and re-enact their past experiences of the Maternal dimensions of existence to help relieve them of their illness and suffering burden. Although there is wide variation in the types of experiences and the types of social roles they recall and dwell on in the Maternal Ground, the centrality of the Maternal to the meaning of their suffering is invariant, and an eidetic structure in all suffering experiences and social relationships for seriously, chronically ill frail and non-frail elderly women and men receiving chronic care. The meaning of the Maternal for these persons is the empathic care they now seek in their vulnerable dependent states, which mirrors, re-enacts and builds upon their passively synthesized experiences of the Maternal. The quest of suffering elders for empathy is a founding, original, and genetic experience rooted in the Maternal Ground. Empathy involves a transposition of self to the vulnerable, dependent other who needs nurturance. Empathy is foundational to the good care that seriously ill persons seek in the care facility from their caregivers.

The home is an essential aspect of the Maternal Ground that is also pervasive in the general structure. The core meanings of the home for elders are multiple— welcome and hospitality, a protective, palliative and pain-free environment, dwelling, inhabiting, nurturance, well-being, and origin. In the absence of the eidetic invariant of the home, the Maternal Ground collapses. Elders' recollections of the comfort and security of the Maternal home motivate the re-enactment of the Maternal system in the care facility in order to create meanings of comfort and security in their struggles living with end-of-life illness. There is an ongoing inimicality between the Maternal home and the anti-Maternal in the realm of suffering that is constantly shifting in the persons' journey through temporal moments of suffering and decision making. At the end of life, persons struggle to recover the lost Maternal Ground and journey toward a Maternal homecoming.

The expanse and depth of these findings about the Maternal and its founding relationship to development and suffering experiences in serious illness and at the end of life are not captured in the literature. While there has been recognition of the role of the Maternal in psychoanalytic treatment (Orange, 2011), in influencing decision making, in schema shaping therapeutic models for treating the seriously ill and dying elders (Parsonnet & Lethoborg, 2011), as well as in care ethics (Roberts & Reich, 2002), there has not been a comprehensive and well thought out integration of the central role and contribution of the Maternal in descriptions and understandings of the social developmental contexts critical to experiences of suffering and decision making. In fact, it is probably more accurate to say that there has been a reluctance to recognize and give the Maternal centrality in these human experiences. The primary and most widely accepted literature on suffering conceptualizes suffering as personal, subjective, and existential in nature (Cassell, 1982, 2004). There is also a body of literature that conceptualizes suffering as having social dimensions (Kleinman & Kleinman, 1997). However, suffering experiences have an intentional structure, and are interpersonal, social, developmental, temporal—with possibilities for agency and self-actualizing.

Agency

Elders' lived experiences of suffering originating in the Maternal Ground have a relationship to agency. There is a constellation of interconnecting relationships in the general structure among agency, spirituality, sociality, and well-being that influences suffering and decision making. Desires for selfhood and independence have a genetic phenomenological structure that is a constituent of the Maternal. The comfort, security, and ongoing care that are given in the Maternal provide the basis for the development of an agentic stance toward the world, an attitude of openness that anticipates limitless possibility – possibility that is delimited by growth, well-being and self-actualizing achievements in the future.

The development of agency is a movement that has temporal dimensions—past, present, and future. There are many different types of agency experienced by older adults in three temporal moments of suffering. The agency before the loss of Maternal Foundations has a different character than the agency that appears as a response to pain and suffering after the loss of Maternal Foundations. Pre-loss agency for seriously ill, elderly women is highly generative, social, and enhanced by perceptions of self-efficacy. Elders experience successes in their enactments, achievements, and engagements in the world—driven in part by their vocational interests. Elderly women and men had rich past lives, experiences, and interests that continued to be present to them in their lives in the care facilities through activation of passively generated and sedimented meanings. For example, Angelique had a "good enough" life in the islands with her mother, but came to the United States, married, worked hard after being widowed, and supported her family. Camila also came to the United States from her native place of origin where she enjoyed a wonderful family life, found a good paying job, married an adoring husband, and continued to serve as the matriarchal head of her extended family. Born in Europe, Josephina came to the United States, married, and was widowed early in life, but worked to support her children and, later in life, her grandchildren, to whom she remained devoted. Harvey, who was a young-old male study participant and a comparison case in the main study, did not experience as much success in his pre-loss life. He led a more marginalized existence both socially and economically, and had a higher level of dependency, weaker perceptions of self-efficacy and a less highly developed spirituality.

Prior to elders' experiences of suffering in care facilities, their agency is located in the Maternal and is associated with flourishing, generativity, and well-being, as discussed above. Elders have loved, formed interpersonal attachments, worked, taken care of others, traveled, and been active members of communities. After being thrown into conditions of pain and suffering in the transition to the care facility environment, and losing Maternal Foundations, elders experience multiple losses and, to varying degrees, some disabling of their agency. However, elders continue to be engaged in many types of agency—practical forms of agency involving use of equipment include eating, toileting, making one's bed, using a walker, and participating in physical therapy. Types of agency that are less related to practical action and evaluation and may be less visible, but involve intentional action for which elders take responsibility and authorship include prayer, seeking empathic care and making appeals to caregivers, engaging in verbal and non-verbal forms of resistance, refusing treatment, and conversation and communication.

In the movement to reconstitute the Maternal Ground and bring it to bear in their current life situations, elderly women and men turn to available resources that foster resilience and recovery of agency as they struggle to cope with their life-limiting and life-threatening conditions. Agency therefore in the third temporal moment becomes a response to pain and suffering that is liberating for them, attempts to lift their burdens of illness and opens up space for them to detach themselves from suffering, and experience self-actualizing in reconstituting the Maternal Ground. Seriously ill elderly persons who undergo care transitions still retain the capacity to be agentic, even in suffering. Suffering does not destroy latent agency or generative capacities to recover from trauma, assaults, and other manifestations of suffering. In suffering, seriously ill elderly women and men may locate agentic resources that coexist in the presence of spirituality.

A great deal of work, research, and writing have been done on agency and what agency means in various contexts in end-of-life illness, planning, and decision making for older adults. Conceptualizations of agency have varied from narrow understandings of intentional action to much broader frameworks of socially and temporally situated enactments and achievements that have cognitive and emotional dimensions. Bandura (1986) developed a social cognitive theory that informs agentic action. Bandura's theory is important because it helps to illuminate how the Maternal is accessible to those who have never experienced the Maternal directly, or have never had positive Maternal experiences or Maternal experiences they can recall with positive feelings. For example, a person who has never been a mother can intuitively apprehend the Maternal.

Similarly, a child who has been treated abusively by a mother may also desire and seek empathic Maternal care and understanding. According to Bandura (1986), other sources of knowledge outside of direct, enactive achievements or failures that inform social cognitive thought are vicarious observations, verbal persuasions, or physiological states of arousal. For elderly women and men who are seriously ill and approaching the end of their lives, it is never too late to experience the Maternal—an issue of significance in their lives in the care facility environment.

Bandura's (1982) work on self-efficacy also has bearing on personal agency as related to seriously ill and frail elders. In a study of the self-efficacy mechanism in human agency, Bandura reported results that demonstrate that perceived self-efficacy helps to explain coping, resignation, and despondency behavior in response to experiences of failure. Sources of self-efficacy information identified by Bandura include enactive achievements, vicarious experiences and observations, verbal persuasion, and physiological states of arousal. This information is processed through cognitive appraisal.

Bandura also cites social and interactive components of self-efficacy.

Gallagher (2007) provides a working definition of agency that is not inconsistent with Bandura's in establishing the distinction between bodily movement and self-agency. According to Gallagher, a sense of agency is not reducible to bodily experience or processes and, therefore, ownership of movement by itself does not constitute self-agency. Gallagher defines agency as an intentional aspect of action, that is, whether the actor is affecting his or her goal and can identify the effect and claim authorship of it.

Emirbayer and Mische (1998) provide a more comprehensive definition which accounts for the temporal and relational aspects of agency:

> a temporally embedded process of social engagement, informed by the past (in its iterational or habitual aspect) but also oriented toward the future (as a projective capacity to imagine alternative possibilities and toward the present as a practical-evaluative capacity to contextualize past habits and future projects within the contingencies of the moment).
>
> (p. 964)

The authors focus on the agentic dimensions of social action as well as the temporal and social aspects of the structures of action.

Agency also needs to be examined with respect to the complexities that arise for persons with dementia. Jennings (2009) elaborates a new relational understanding of agency for persons with dementia that moves away from conceptualizing agency in purely hedonic terms. This reframing of agency illuminates Husserl's natural attitude—the attitude of the taken-for-granted everyday world—in that it is not the same for everyone. Persons with dementia are in a natural attitude that is radically different from the natural attitude of persons with capacity.

Important work has also been done on expanding the concept of agency in older adults with diminished capacities and dementias (Jennings, 2009). Agency in these narratives reveals itself as multifaceted expressions of the self in the process of human development. That process takes in experiences of suffering as well as other experiences of meaning to elderly women and men approaching the end of life. Meanings are not determined by health, but are created in varying stages of the life course even at the end of life and in liminal states and are valued by seriously ill elderly persons. The narratives help to illuminate the relationship of agency to constituents of suffering and agentic processes of decision making and self-actualizing at the end of life, and show that agency plays a prominent role in the social development of suffering and decision making and can be a palliative response to suffering.

Sociality

Sociality and social systems are salient in the general structure of suffering. There is a relationship among agency, sociality, spirituality, and suffering. Elderly women and men are embedded in social systems in their lives in chronic care facilities. The research findings and narratives suggest that sociality is the fabric that undergirds life in care facilities, even in the midst of suffering. There is a web of social and interpersonal connections and relationships across social systems—personal, family, caregiver, interdisciplinary team, care facility—that is not vitiated by suffering experiences. Even elders who express feelings of loneliness are reflecting a need for social connection and a lack of meaningful relationship with others. Empathy, one of the core constituents of the Maternal that founds social life, is pervasive among frail elders in care facilities and occurs at pre-reflective levels. Many elderly women and men in the care facilities demonstrate empathic care and concern for each other in meaningful ways—such as active listening when one is in need of having intimate conversation, assisting in practical tasks such as making telephone calls to reach loved ones, assisting those who are non-ambulatory, and providing emotional support to each other upon loss of a fellow resident.

These relationships among systems have a deep meaning for the frail elders. Pain and suffering experiences themselves are fundamentally social and relational. The interembodied social character of life in the Maternal is re-enacted by elders in their experiences in the care facilities, even in their suffering. The loss of Maternal Foundations does not completely isolate the social and relational dimensions and meanings of pain and suffering experiences for elders. While the constituents of suffering are very much associated with experiences of loss—including loss of sociality—suffering persons are situated in a social world and within social contexts within which they are having ongoing interactions. Research shows that loneliness may be concerned with the strength of the quality of relationships and the deficiency of sociality more than its absence altogether (Cacioppo & Patrick, 2008; Dumm, 2008; Hawkley et al., 2008). Loneliness is still a mode of sociality. Suffering persons themselves have emotional responses to suffering that are apprehended by others, and their emotional responses as well as the responses of their relational others have implications for the trajectory of the suffering experience. There is increasingly a focus on the role of the emotions in social experiences of pain and suffering (Cagle & Altilio, 2011; Morrissey, 2011a, 2011b; Nussbaum, 2001). John Drummond's (2008a) work in moral phenomenology, which gives a clear portrait of how the emotions are involved in valuing and in becoming fully responsible moral agents, can be brought to bear in understanding the role of emotions and valuing in suffering experience. The capacity to be agentic and to create and renew social connections opens up opportunities for self-actualization and self-acceptance, recovery and resilience. Suffering by virtue of its very structure involves locating suffering persons in their social worlds and in their developmental social contexts.

Sociality also has meaning for elders as members of communities. There is the community within the facilities and the community outside them, and an ongoing tension between these two realms. Prior to the loss of Maternal Foundations, elders are members of communities at varying levels of agency and in many different domains—work, religion, family life, music, culture, socioeconomic production and consumption, urban life. Elders share some commonality in belonging to an urban community where there is socioeconomic disadvantage. The loss of Maternal dimensions involves to some extent a loss of community. In transitioning to care facilities, elders are relocated to a new community where they develop new social roles and relationships with their caregivers and health care professionals and other residents. But there continues to be a nexus between the community in the care facility and the community outside the facility. Elders such as Angelique and Harvey are aware of their continuing disadvantage with limited resources and relying on government programs for their health care. The relationship between elders' place in the external community, the urban neighborhood environment and its social determinants, and the experience of suffering survives care transitions and the move to the facility.

Spirituality

Spirituality, the third central system resting on the Maternal Ground, interacts with agency and sociality and has meaning for elders in their suffering and decision-making experiences. Spirituality manifests itself as springs from the Maternal—and in some instances as an expression of agency in the first temporal moment. Spirituality is itself a ground for the possibility of recovery and resilience in the second and third temporal moments of suffering. The founding relationships of the Maternal to agency, sociality and spirituality, and the relationship of spirituality and agency to suffering and decision making are significant social structures for seriously, chronically ill elderly women and men living in care facility communities.

Spirituality, in the lives of elders, is a pervasive system that grounds and coexists with suffering. The quest for meaning and for a connectedness that transcends self becomes even more important for elders whose life-worlds are threatened by serious and life-limiting illness. Spirituality is a source of strength for elders during their suffering and enables agency. Conversely, agency can also enable and strengthen spirituality.

Second Temporal Moment: Vortex of Pain and Suffering

Loss of Maternal Foundations by elders thrusts them into a vortex of pain— bodily, emotional, and social. In transitioning to the care facility, elders are displaced from their homes and experience the trauma of dislocation, of being transplanted to a new environment that is foreign to them and threatening to their comfort and security. They descend into a shrunken spatiality and temporality and have little access to the relational intimacy with family members and caregivers that they had prior to the dislocation. One of the major losses suffering elders may sustain in this period is the loss or disabling of agency—loss of independence, loss of control, loss of autonomy, loss of bodily function and of corporeality itself, loss of meaning, loss of self, loss of dignity, and loss of full participation in decision making. However, there is variation in the experience of agency and diminution of agency. Some elders have more agentic capacity than others. In the narrative data analyses, Harvey, who was a younger older adult with complex wounds receiving chronic care, has a much more disabled agency than the seriously ill elderly women and other men in the facilities.

These losses and traumas coexist with the experience of bodily pain that sometimes begins with the experience of frailty, as in the case of Angelique. Elders experience frailty as bodily weakness, loss of energy, and general weakness of the lower extremities. Frailty opens elders to the assaults of multiple comorbidities and a trajectory toward serious, chronic illness and end of life. Elders in the studies had multiple chronic illnesses involving multiple systems—such as congestive heart failure, coronary artery disease, advanced peripheral vascular disease, diabetes, and kidney dysfunction—and were in varying stages of frailty, multimorbidity, and declining health trajectories.

Phenomenologically, pain is not reducible to a bodily experience alone. It has multiple structural, process, and outcome dimensions. Pain is usually a sensory experience felt within the body, such as the pain Angelique had in her hands and feet from her Parkinson's disease. But pain may also be taken up as feelings—bodily feelings and emotional responses. All of the elders have powerful responses to their pain across a range of emotions—anger, shame, fear.

The emotional structure of pain has complexity and involves an evaluation of the pain experience. Elders value, or attach value attributes, to their pain experiences. This valuing has social and relational dimensions, as elders are situated in social environments and have interpersonal relationships that shape their responses to pain.

The conceptualization of pain that emerges from elders' descriptions originates in most cases with a sensory, bodily experience to which there is a two-fold—bodily and emotional—response (Morrissey, 2011a). In some cases, however, pain is not associated with any tissue damage and may be the result of suffering. In the social context of family, facility environments, and other systems, elders' pain also demands a response from health care professionals, caregivers, and relational others. Their responses affect and influence the course of the pain experience and the emotional dimensions of pain. There is variation in elders' emotional responses based upon the management of the pain. If pain is not appropriately managed, feelings of anxiety, frustration, and diminished self-efficacy may contribute to an escalation of pain and cultivate heightened emotional responses. Pain is a social and relational system involving dialectical process interactions, with the self and others, that change over time.

There are important implications of these findings for assessment and treatment of pain for seriously ill elderly persons. First, pain is not reducible to a medical outcome. It is a process that calls for more sophisticated and person-centered types of assessments. Relying on the elder's report is of course well established—if the elder is able to report. But the complexity of assessment involving social context and systems is not well recognized. It is important for social work practitioners, in particular, to sort out the role and influence of each system—personal, family, delivery, and others—and the cognitive, affective, and interpersonal dimensions of pain experiences.

The social work literature on pain, as well as pain and symptom management, has focused on these important aspects of the pain problem for seriously ill individuals: the ethical obligation of social workers to respond to pain; the need to understand the complexity and scope of pain as a multidimensional presenting problem; the importance of multidimensional assessment of pain; and the need to develop a stronger evidence base for effective social work interventions to relieve pain (Cagle & Altilio, 2011). Fostering interdisciplinary practice and elimination of barriers to appropriate pain care for minority and marginalized populations are also important goals for all of the helping professions. These goals take on critical priority for seriously ill elderly women and men, especially in resource-poor urban care facilities where they count among the most vulnerable and marginalized individuals in society. Considerably more work and investments of resources need to be made in studying and understanding chronic pain, its unique trajectories, pathways, and relationship to older adults' social ecology of health and well-being.

Suffering and its social developmental contexts

All of the elders in the research studies experienced suffering in the care facility environment during their end-of-life illness. Suffering is not a monolithic, seamless experience for these elders. Suffering is a changing and complex social developmental structure that is rooted in the Maternal dimensions of experience and has agentic, emotional, and other dimensions. Suffering manifests itself in a number of different ways, including as a structural, social process involving social systems and actors; a pervasive threat to every aspect of experience; a shock, trauma, or fall from height; dislocation, displacement, or alienation; oppression, marginalization, or branding; victimization; voicelessness; vulnerability; dependency; losses of autonomy, self, role, dignity, humanity, and meaning; accumulation of burden; affliction, no relief or rescue; and threat to futural horizon. One elderly person described her suffering as not being associated with a loss of meaning, but with emptiness, the darkness of night and desolation of the desert. In many instances, language lacks the capacity to express fully the meanings of suffering for frail elders. In such circumstances, eidetic phenomenological analysis of suffering experience that is at a pre-conceptual and pre-verbal level allows intuitive grasping of the essence of suffering through the systematic process of exemplification and imaginative variation, as done in these research studies. What is invariant in suffering experience is pervasive unbounded and indeterminate losses of Maternal Foundations and agency. These pervasive losses of Maternal Foundations and agency are present in all examples of suffering and all possibilizing of suffering, and therefore, are at a high level generality.

For example, Angelique experiences suffering in perceiving a "chicken head" on her lunch plate. The meaning of this experience for her is that she is stigmatized as less than human and without dignity. She experiences the care facility environment as oppressive and feels herself a victim. She has strong emotional responses to the dislocation, stigmatization and marginalization she experiences, and to the associated losses of Maternal Foundations; she is angry and ashamed, and values the experiences negatively.

Camila suffers terribly when she is drawn into an incident with another resident because of a cultural miscommunication that Camila understood to be derisive of a cultural icon of the Maternal. The meaning of the Maternal for Camila is so sacred that her emotional response exceeds normative behavior: she hits the other resident. This cascades into a series of consequences for Camila that compound her suffering and losses, and weaken her self-efficacy and agency.

Josephina's suffering arises from the burdens of her chronic illnesses: bodily pains and discomforts from her disabling edematous conditions and medications, waiting endlessly to be taken care of by the staff, and the terrible emotional anguish she experiences when she cannot control her bodily functions. Her loss of control and functioning, and illness burden, prevent her from attending the funeral service of her friend who has passed away.

The meanings of suffering for Harvey and Ruth appear as loss of agency. Harvey is halted in time and space by his disabling condition. His emotional responses to his disabilities heighten his suffering and impair his coping mechanisms. Ruth also struggles with lost agency in the care facility. She shares that she is no longer able to sing the way she once did. Singing was her life and the center of her social life. The meaning of this loss of song reflects her dislocation and displacement, and her voicelessness in the care facility.

Ann suffers from a serious respiratory illness, but she turns to smoking for the empathic comfort and security of the Maternal that she cannot locate from her caregivers in the care facility. She describes an experience of being told by the care facility staff that she can no longer receive physical therapy services because she is "nasty". She feels that she has been pegged as undeserving and calls upon her son to intervene on her behalf. But she finds nurture in a circle of residents who congregate every day in the garden to smoke.

The complexities involved in losses of Maternal Foundations and agency are such, however, that elders' vulnerability and dependency in care facilities do not assure permanent losses of the Maternal dimensions of existence and agency. Frail and non-frail elderly persons sometimes have changing moods and declining mental health status, but they retain a capacity to be agentic. They may seek relational, empathic care, although they may not be communicative in the ways that have been expected of them in the past.

Patient Decision Making at End of Life

Elders are engaged in various types of decision making in care facilities. Decision making is a process that concerns the elder and decisions about the elder's care—from health care and treatment decisions to other types of decisions such as choice of community. Decision making has multidimensional attributes: cognitive, affective, social, communicative, relational, and evaluative. Elders attach value attributes to their decisions—such as "good" or "bad." Decision making can also be collaborative and shared, to the extent that it involves persons other than elders—health care agents, family members, and health care professionals.

Elders engage in end-of-life decision making as a form of agency as they move into a third temporal moment of adapting to their serious and life-limiting illnesses. Decision making is a response to suffering. Elders make different types of decisions—from the routine to life-sustaining treatment decisions. Decision making involves a temporal process of choosing between alternatives: weighing risks, burdens, and benefits, and engaging in meaningful communication with caregivers and health care professionals.

Relationships with health care professionals are an important factor in decision making for frail elders residing in care facilities. However, trusted family members are even more important than health care professionals.

Temporal, Developmental, and Genetic Aspects of Suffering

Suffering as it appeared in the lived experiences of frail elders had a temporal and developmental horizonality. Stone and Papadimitriou (2011) have identified three "equiprimordial" moments or "ecstasies" in Heidegger's temporality: "having been, making present, and the future, none of which exist *in* time, but all of which, experienced together allow us to *exist as* temporal beings" (p. 138). Charmaz (1997) and Cassell (1982) have recognized temporality as an important dimension of illness. Therefore, the conceptualizations of illness experience and illness burden in this study as having temporal dimensions are not new, but build on widely accepted phenomenological analyses and humanistic understandings of temporality.

Eric J. Cassell (1982), a physician who made seminal contributions to our understanding of suffering, wrote almost three decades ago that suffering has temporal elements. In his work 'The Nature of Suffering and the Goals of Medicine', Cassell (1982) discussed how persons who are suffering have changing perceptions of their future in struggling with fears and anxieties about the unknown and death. Cassell also acknowledged the role of past experiences, including illness experiences and the role of culture and other factors, in shaping suffering experiences. The temporal moments of suffering identified in this study expand upon, and in some instances depart from, Cassell's descriptions of the temporal elements of suffering.

This study describes three temporal moments of suffering and the experiences and meanings that are invariant in each temporal moment for seriously ill elderly women and men. The flow of the moments is iterative and plastic—depending upon the course of development. The descriptions of the three temporal moments also ground temporality in a Maternal origin upon which suffering experiences are founded and are dependent. The Maternal as origin is an archeological site and wellspring of resources for vulnerable elderly persons who access the givens of the Maternal in recollections—building up passive syntheses of past experiences that are activated in these recollections. Phenomenological methods provide access to these temporal moments of suffering and reveal them as part of a unitary structure of suffering or whole. These moments are not separate and distinct elements or parts of suffering experiences, but are moments in a horizon that has a genetic origin and is a referential framework for actual experiences that have already become present—as well as past experiences that have been passively generated and limitless unknown experiences in the future (Geniusas, 2010). Geniusas (2010) discusses his conceptualization of the horizon as a "system of reference and a system of validity" (p. 82) and its meaning in terms of origin. The horizon is referential in that it takes in all appearances, and valid because potential modes of appearance are contained within actual appearances. According to Geniusas (2010), origin is the origin of the horizon. These genetic notions of horizon and origin have meaning for the structures of suffering and decision making. Suffering is a horizon that has an origin and a horizonality that implicates the lived past and future in the present. Turning attention to suffering experiences in the present requires understanding the role of the past and possibilities for the future in the present.

Cassell also discussed the flow of time in terms of the relationship of suffering to the present and the future. He states: "…suffering would not exist in the absence of a future" (Cassell, 2004, p. 35). The narratives reveal meanings of seriously ill older adults that run counter to this interpretation of suffering as personalized and amenable to the control of the person in the present moment. Rather, it is in the excruciating immediacy of the present that elders experience unbearable suffering. Recollection and re-enactment of the lived past, and imagining and envisioning a future act to relieve suffering. Departing from Cassell (1999) in his restriction of suffering to the sphere of the personal and that which belongs only to the individual, the phenomenological concept of horizon permits an understanding of the horizon of suffering that is broader than the personal or individual and includes the social world intersubjectively experienced by persons. Geniusas (2010) identified world experience as a phenomenological level of the horizon. While Cassell clearly identifies the multiple social, cultural, familial, and lived past dimensions and meanings of personhood, he remains committed to a conceptualization of suffering that is personal and individual only. Husserl (1989), who has advanced phenomenological methods in psychology, developed a concept of inner time consciousness which describes the past, present, and future dimensions of temporality. The findings in these narratives about the temporality of suffering build on phenomenological understandings of the horizon and inner time consciousness. The narratives demonstrate that the suffering experiences of seriously ill elderly women and men are not isolated events in time. The current experiences of elderly women and men in the present have social contexts that draw upon their past experiences. In a first temporal moment of lived experience, the social context of suffering is a previous life with family and community that has been built on Maternal Foundations. The narratives disclose the often rich personal histories of frail elders who are spending the last months of their lives in care facilities and their recollections of past experiences in their current situatedness in such facilities. These foundations, and the social life built on them, are lost in the process of suffering in a central moment of care transitions that leads elderly women and men into care facility environments where they continue to live through such losses. The retained experience of the Maternal is what these very sick women and men sought to re-establish in the care facilities in a third temporal moment in relations with caregivers, family members and other residents, as a reconstituted ground for recovered agency and spiritual well-being, and as a remedy for the losses they have suffered. The transcendence or relief of suffering in the facility environment depends on the successful re-establishment of Maternal care, Maternal relations, and a welcoming home that supports the personal growth, recovery and reactivation of agency, and achievement of well-being. The narratives also show how the suffering experiences of elderly women and men shape their visions and imaginative variations of the future.

Genetic approach to human development and formation of interpersonal attachments

In studying the experiences of suffering, seriously ill, and often frail elderly women and men at the end of life, it is important to understand how suffering experiences develop and influence elderly persons' life course even at the end of their lives. Based upon the literature, this may be described as a genetic approach to human development (Bandura, 1977, 1986, 1997; Barber, 2011; Geniusas, 2011; Guntrip, 1973).[1] This approach expands upon Freud's (1930) psychoanalytic work on early Maternal–child relations and child development and the work of others who followed him—such as Piaget (1932), Erikson (1950), and Winnicott (1965). Merleau-Ponty (1964) also explored these issues in *The Child's Relations with Others* in the context of an intercorporeal schema or "system" that is essential to perception (p. 117). Bandura (1977, 1986, 1997) adopted a developmental approach to the investigation and understanding of social cognitive learning and self-efficacy which departs from psychodynamic theory, but retains strong social developmental elements of understanding human behavior. This approach recognized the interaction of personal and social systems in the environment in the development of agency and self-efficacy. Phenomenologists building on the work of Husserl have turned to genetic phenomenology to address questions of origin—such as the horizon (Geniusas, 2010) and the development of empathy (Barber, 2010). Ira Byock (2002) in his work and writing on the "meaning and value of death" recognized the role of development and personal growth in coming to grips with death.

These narratives identify developmental aspects of suffering that expand upon well-established research in human development. Guntrip (1973) discusses at length the evolution of knowledge, beginning with Freud (1930), on the development of selfhood through the processes of interpersonal relating and human attachment. According to Guntrip, this process of development cannot be conflated or confused with biologically oriented conceptualizations of adaptation to the environment. Guntrip's discussion and analysis drew heavily on work done by Winnicott on the emotional development of infants from the time of birth and the Maternal role in ego-relatedness in the mature person. Guntrip focuses on the meaning of a self in relationship with others that is not delimited by transactions with the environment or a mere drive to survive. DeRobertis (2010), also drawing upon Winnicott, advanced a social developmental perspective on well-being that is rooted in early child development and what he described as "good enough" mothering. DeRobertis described an interpersonal facilitating environment in which the primary caregiver engages in activities of holding and handling which are essential to the development of a sense of well-being in the child. Two key constituents of these mothering activities are empathy, or a putting oneself in the place of the baby, and identification—a shifting of a sense of self to the baby (DeRobertis, 2010). Merleau-Ponty (1964) also recognized this process of the child's identification in the Maternal relation through experiencing, assimilating, and role-playing. According to DeRobertis, the constituents and characteristics of an empathic, responsive, and facilitating environment that encourage strong ego development lay a foundation for self-actualization and the formation of interpersonal attachments he described as innate drivers of early child development. Researchers have recognized the role of attachment and attachment anxiety in the care-seeking behavior of older adults (Karantzas, Evans, & Foddy, 2010).

Two theorists who focused on self-actualization in human development were Maslow (1954), who elaborated a theory based upon a hierarchy of human needs, and Rogers (1961) who suggested that human development is a process involving self-acceptance, openness to experience, and empathic understanding. These theories share ground with psychoanalytic developmental theories in conceptualizing self-actualization as involving more than simply need gratification. Guntrip (1973) used the example of the infant whose hunger can be satisfied through nursing, but who still desires to suckle at the mother's breast because of the need to be in a relationship with the mother. According to Guntrip, Winnicott described these intense relational experiences as non-climactic and non-orgiastic, distinguishing them from climactic satisfaction of instinctual, orgiastic experiences. DeRobertis's descriptions of Maternal–infant and early child development in his elaboration of the essential activities of maternal holding and integration that respond to the ontological demands of the infant or child, or frail elder, to the child confirm the significance of the social and relational aspects of development.

Merleau-Ponty's (1964) work in *The Child's Relations with Others* perhaps best describes phenomenologically what he calls syncretic sociability or the non-differentiated state in a Maternal holding environment that a baby shares with its mother in early childhood development. Merleau-Ponty's work makes certain important contributions to the understanding of sociality in development and its critical relevance to seriously ill elderly persons at the end of life. First, Merleau-Ponty debunked what he called classical thinking and misconceptions about the psyche being inaccessible by others and accessible only to oneself, and described the way in which consciousness is disclosed in the world through the way in which one interacts with the world in one's conduct. Merleau-Ponty (1964) states, "my consciousness is turned primarily toward the world, turned toward things; it is above all a relation to the world" (p. 117). Merleau-Ponty (1964) elaborates further on this fundamental social relation by describing consciousness of the body as a "postural schema" that locates the position of the body as a "system" in relation to the environment (p. 117). This is very much along the lines of what is revealed in these narratives in terms of the postural stance in the Maternal relation for seriously ill elderly women and men. However, according to Merleau-Ponty, prior to the development of consciousness of the body, an ego, and the formation of a self, the infant or child in the syncretic state has no awareness of the other as separate or different or as having a separate body, and is in an anonymous, undifferentiated state of collectivity. In this description of intercorporeality and the genesis of consciousness, the child's first and original relations with the world are in the Maternal relation with the mother's breast. Zaner (2002) echoes the view of the Maternal as an original experience that has relevance to later life development in his analysis of Schütz's "We-relation", as well as others who discuss the meaning of birth and breastfeeding (Ryan et al., 2010; Simms, 2001; Wertz, 1981). From the very beginning, we are with the other, as Zaner explains Schütz's perspective on intersubjectivity (2002). This is a primordial, genetic experience that is retained forever in the life history of each human person, and establishes a Maternal Ground for sociality, agency and spirituality over the life course.

In order to understand the primordial, genetic experience of the Maternal Ground fully, it is necessary to make the transcendental turn in phenomenology as explained in Chapter 1. The transcendental *epoché* gives access to the constituting "I" of consciousness. In the transcendental reduction, the world is bracketed. The transcendental lens shows how the Maternal Ground is socially constituted through actual experience and then later through passively synthesized meanings that are built up over the life course. These meanings are sedimented in our social worlds and social and cultural life, and form the basis for active generation of meanings. In the intentional structure of consciousness, suffering is an actively generated meaning that involves losses of Maternal Foundations and agency that are located in the pre-reflective, common sense world. Suffering is a loss of passivity—a loss of the passively generated meanings that implicate the futural horizon and all future meaningful activity that presuppose passivity. At the transcendental level, suffering is the severing or collapse of the intentional relation with the world, or subject-world correlation, and the isolation of consciousness and subjectivity from the objective world of meanings. It is the negation of all the meanings of the Maternal: presence, corporeality, availability, generativity. But subjectivity can rescue itself from its exile because it can generate new meanings and can recover the social world.

The descriptions of the Maternal as original and syncretic, that show up at other times in one's life course, have relevance for seriously ill elderly persons. Frail elders who are burdened with chronic illness re-enact the syncretic experience of being with the other in the Maternal relation in the care facility environment. Merleau-Ponty calls this transitivism, and says it manifests itself as an attribution to others of what the subject is experiencing or authoring. In making a parallel to Piaget's notion of displacement and the retention of syncretism at higher levels of development, Merleau-Ponty (1964) explains, "syncretic sociability can be found in the sick to the extent to which they regress in the direction of the conduct of children and show themselves incapable of making the transition to praxis to the selfless outgoing attitude of the adult" (p. 155). The seriously ill women and men in this study recollect past experiences of the Maternal in an attempt to reactivate the comfort, empathy, and security of Maternal care to help relieve their suffering in care facilities. This re-enactment may go through developmental stages of regression, but the development as a whole is part of the life-drive of frail elders as they strive to recover agency.

The role of the Maternal in the development of the suffering experiences of seriously ill elderly women and men is primary and originary in nature and influences the evolution of suffering over the life course through the three temporal moments. The developmental aspects of suffering are inseparable from the social and interpersonal experiences of frail elders living in care facilities and the formation of their identity and reconstitution of self at the end of their lives.

Cassell (2004) has recognized the social aspects of suffering experiences in his description of social roles, consciousness of others, interpersonal relationships, and the affective dimensions of such relationships. However, the elaboration of the social developmental aspects of suffering seems to go beyond what Cassell is willing to acknowledge as within the legitimate boundaries of suffering as experienced by persons. Cassell (2004) makes clear in his exegesis on suffering that "suffering is experienced by persons" (p. 127), is not limited to the body, the mind, the spiritual, or that which is "only subjectively knowable" (p. 127). According to Cassell, suffering is as complex as personhood itself in all its variegated dimensions. In his conclusions, however, Cassell holds unwaveringly to the notion that suffering is personal, and while related to any dimension of the person, "is ultimately a personal matter" (p. 128).

The chapter narratives are consistent with certain aspects of what Cassell has so well described as the nature of suffering. Elderly women and men struggling with life-limiting and life-threatening illness experience suffering, as persons and as developed over the life course. Suffering therefore is experienced in lived time and lived space. However, Cassell's limitation of the nature of suffering to a personal matter is itself too limited. Yes, suffering has shared meanings, as Cassell acknowledges. But there is something more complex going on: the essentially social nature of suffering. Adopting the social developmental perspective that comes out of psychoanalysis and developmental psychology, as well as social cognitive theory, social ecology and social work—seriously ill elderly women and men living in care facilities, or wherever they may be situated, are persons in environment. Sociality is the very ground of their intentionalities, consciousness, and agency, even in their suffering experiences. Using imaginative variation, it is not possible to conceive of a person with a developed or developing self who never experienced social connection. The life-worlds of seriously ill elderly women and men who are suffering are intersubjectively experienced and socially constituted. The narratives reveal that the person's experience of suffering from its very beginning is fundamentally interpersonal, social, and relational because individuation of consciousness and formation of the self are processes that follow the primordial process of being joined together. The process of suffering implicates what psychologist David Bakan (1968) described in his essay on pain, suffering and disease as the "social telos" from which the suffering person becomes isolated, and the "telic decentralization" of the organizing systems of the self (p. 47). This social telos described by Bakan is located in the primordial Maternal Ground. The social foundations and agency that constitute decentralizing losses for suffering elders may be restored through reactivation and re-enactment of the Maternal.

Meanings of the Maternal Ground for Seriously Ill Elders

The research findings of empathic care that appeared in the lives of frail elders in the care facilities resonates with discussions about the meaning of an ethic of care in the body of sociological and feminist writings on embodied care (Hamington, 2004), and a feminist ethic of care that draws upon Merleau-Ponty, as well as the early social work pioneers Jane Addams and Mary Richmond, and psychologist Carol Gilligan (1993). Hammond (2004) described the role of imagination in empathy as "transcend[ing] both physics and social distance to help create the potential for care through empathy" (p. 69). Hamington cited and credited Merleau-Ponty for establishing by implication, in his phenomenological descriptions of the body and intercorporeality, the pervasiveness of empathy in the "continuity of the flesh" (p. 69).

Sympathy, relationality, interpersonal holism, embodiment, voice, agency, "consociates," the Maternal, and empathy are all aspects of an ethic of care identified by Mary Rogers (2009), and Gilligan. According to Gilligan, an ethic of care pre-empts an ethic of rights. Gilligan (1993) suggests that attachment and responsibility in relationships are more meaningful for the psychological development of women than a gendered preoccupation with autonomy, right and the individual. This perspective on a relational paradigm in care ethics is gaining prominence in the public discourse about the person- and family-centered palliative ethic of care (Fins, 2006), and the relation-centered process interactions involved in end-of-life decision making (Morrissey & Jennings, 2006). The implications of the relational paradigm emerging in palliative and end-of-life care in a movement away from more dominant medical and formalistic frameworks of decision making were explored by Morrissey (2011a) in a descriptive account of the phenomenology of pain and suffering experiences for older adults and the role of the emotions in such experiences. Elders desire meaningful relationships with their caregivers and with family members as they struggle and cope with their suffering and illness burden.

The home is an essential aspect of the Maternal Ground. The core meanings of the home are multiple: welcome and hospitality, protective environment, dwelling, inhabiting, nurturance, well-being, and origin. In the absence of the eidetic invariant of the home, the Maternal Ground would collapse. The metaphor of the Maternal as home and welcoming hospitality has been used by Levinas in his description of a relational ethics as responsibility to the other. The findings of this study confirm Levinas's (1969) conceptualization of the Maternal as being essentially social and ethical in character.

The Maternal call or invocation is an ethical claim that seriously ill elderly women and men make upon their caregivers to provide appropriate empathic care to them in their states of dependency. There is an ongoing inimicality between the home as having the meaning of the Maternal and the meaning of the anti-Maternal as threat and alienation in a realm of suffering outside the home. This tension between "homelike" and "unhomelike" was constantly in shift in the elders' journey through temporal moments of suffering and decision making. The experience of threat was pervasive among the participants in their experiences of care transitions to facilities in the first temporal moment of suffering. At the end of life, elders struggled to recover the lost Maternal Ground and journeyed toward a Maternal homecoming. What did this homecoming mean for participants?

Dekkers (2001), writing for the Pallium research project in Europe, provided the most comprehensive description and understanding of the meanings of the home. He discussed the home in the context of origin and returning to roots, the character of the home environment as welcoming or "homelike" or its antithesis, the relationship of the home to health, and the "coming home" journey at the end of life. The findings of my research studies confirmed many of the meanings of home elaborated on by Dekkers as they relate to the goals of palliative care. The home appears as origin in the sense of where one's life and development began, as discussed previously, and appealed to participants as a return to their roots at the end of life.

The home also manifests itself as a felt sense of well-being and a process of finding one's way back home. Dekkers (2001) discussed existential meanings of the home as being in a "homelike" world in the Heideggerian sense, consistent with the phenomenological approach of Bernd Jager (1979) and Merleau-Ponty (1964) to understanding the lived body as housedness and dwelling, and a form of operative intentionality in and toward the world. The literature Dekkers drew upon conceptualized health as "homelike"—escaping the trauma of being homeless in living with serious illness. While notions of health as freedom from pain, suffering and trauma fit the ideal of the Maternal as absolute welcome, intertwining and interembodiment, the Maternal homecoming in the third temporal moment involves suffering in the presence of a desire for well-being, agentic purpose and action, and spiritual meanings. The horizon of suffering appeared as a vista—an opening up of a space for self-actualizing—even at the end of life. This description of elders' journey at the end of life as "coming home" or "homecoming" has an eidetic meaning that was related to the Maternal. Participants' homecoming involves a movement toward a final place of rest, an imagined future that holds the possibility of hope and spiritual well-being at the end of life.

In addition, Dekkers (2001) discussed existential meanings of the home as being-in-the-world. Dekkers drew upon conceptualizations of the "homelike" that framed it as the equivalence of health or, according to his own notion, relief from suffering. Dekkers was not entirely correct. The structure of a Maternal homecoming in the third temporal moment of the structure of suffering is not delimited by health or relief from suffering alone. Instead, participants oftentimes navigate through experiences of suffering in the presence of a desire for well-being, agentic purpose, action, and spiritual meanings. The horizon of suffering presents limitless opportunities for self-actualizing—even at the end of life.

While frail elders living in the care facilities demonstrated the capacity to assimilate meanings of the Maternal and empathic care, and to accommodate changes in their personal and social systems, one young-old male participant had weakened agentic capacity in the face of terrible illness burden. This particular person had experienced a partial amputation of his leg, and had also had a prior life of hardship and suffering. Significantly, his spiritual foundations were not as highly developed as other elderly persons. However, even as this study-participant struggled with a collapsed agency similar to the rupture or breakdown in temporal existence described previously by Stone and Papadimitriou (2011), he continued to communicate his desires for well-being and social connection, and to imagine a future in which he would no longer be totally dependent on others. He experienced the nursing home as a Maternal system of care replacing his lost Maternal Foundations.

The expanse and depth of these findings in regard to the role and meanings of the Maternal in end-of-life illness and decision making are not captured adequately in the gerontological and social work literature. Early work in psychoanalysis and by those who followed including Erikson (1950) and Winnicott (1965), certainly lay important foundations for working with seriously ill elderly persons and their families. The primary and most widely accepted work conceptualizes suffering as essentially personal and individual in nature (Cassell, 1999). Cassell has discussed the diagnosis of suffering and the need for physicians to learn to work with subjective information about the suffering person including evidence of disease and symptoms. Many of Cassell's recommendations for recognizing and engaging in dialogue with persons about their suffering have greatly advanced the state of knowledge about human suffering, its assessment, and treatment. However, even given Cassell's (1999) strong focus on the nature of suffering as an "affliction of persons," he appears to remain embedded—although his typology of personhood would suggest otherwise—in a medical model of diagnosis and syndrome identification, restricting his rich understanding of personhood to the personal, individual, and subjective without integrating such understanding with knowledge of the intersubjectively experienced social world of suffering persons. There is a strong countering body of literature that conceptualizes suffering as having multi-level social dimensions, including both social interactions that are central to illness experience and collective experiences that influence the development and trajectory of suffering. Anthropologists Kleinman and Kleinman (1997) problematize approaches to suffering that pathologize and commercialize suffering, victimize sufferers, and attempt to measure suffering in terms of utilitarian metrics of economic cost and efficiency. The authors call for a re-evaluation of indexes of individual suffering that overlook social modes of suffering and a recentering on local and interpersonal space in lieu of distanced policy perspectives and stances for viewing suffering (Kleinman & Kleinman, 1997). Kleinman and Kleinman also jettison artificial distinctions between the health and social aspects of suffering, and individual and social lenses on suffering experience. Suffering has a complex intentional structure encompassing interpersonal, social, developmental, and temporal contexts. Suffering's essential constituents and invariant eidetic meanings constitute a unitary whole that is located in a social world. Previous treatments of suffering have focused on partial views and analyses of suffering experiences that do not take full account of the intersubjectively-experienced social world in which seriously ill, elderly persons live and develop, even at the end of life. In view of my strivings through this project to recover the social worlds of suffering, I draw on Schütz's concept of an "enclave" to help illuminate these social world of suffering in which agency, sociality and spirituality share lived space.

Enclave of Agency, Sociality, and Spirituality in Suffering and Decision Making: Agency as Expression of Resilience

Elders' lived experiences of suffering, originating in the Maternal Ground, relate to agency. There is a constellation, or "enclave" as Schütz described it (Schutz, 1962/1973; Rogers, 2008), of interconnecting relationships in the general structure among agency, spirituality, sociality, and well-being that influence suffering and decision making. Mary Rogers (2009) describes Schütz's enclaves as "intensely lived experiences of multiple realities" (p. 14). The constituents of suffering that rest on the Maternal Ground share the characteristics of being phenomenologically distinct but often overlapping realms of experience and shared lived space for seriously ill elderly women and men. Desire for selfhood and independence has a genetic phenomenological structure that is constitutive of the Maternal. The comfort, security, and ongoing care that are given in the Maternal provide the basis for the development of an agentic stance toward the world: an attitude of openness that anticipates limitless possibility and self-actualizing achievements in the future. The development of agency is also a movement that has temporal dimensions—past, present, and future.

Policy Implications

The narratives present significant policy issues. The structure of suffering is generalized to seriously, chronically ill women and men residing in care facilities.

The findings of this study are consistent with the literature on seriously, chronically ill elderly women and men, and their social and medical profile both generally and in care facilities providing chronic care. The participants in the narratives ranged in age from the young-old to 96—three women and four men in the follow up study, and six women and two men in the original study. Overall, five men of a total of 15 participants in the narratives had complex, chronic wounds. All of the participating elders had multiple chronic illnesses. This portrait of the study-participants provides evidence of dependency.

All of these elders are burdened with serious illness and chronicity, and multiple limitations in activities of daily living. The literature establishes a relationship between disability, frailty, and a compressed dying trajectory. The narratives suggest that there is such a relationship between the burdens of chronic illness, disability, and frailty and the course of illness and dying.

Seriously ill elderly women and men are facing ever-growing complex social, health, and economic needs that define their dependency on social welfare programs with shrinking economic resources. Dependency for older adults is not a given and, to some extent, may be socially constructed by society and institutions, and by older adults themselves (Cox, 2005). Patterns of medicalization and commodification contribute to the marginalization of older adults within society and exacerbate their dependency needs. In light of growth of chronic illness burden, longer life expectancies, and higher risk for impoverishment (Berkman et al., 2006), the dependency problem for elderly women is magnified.

The social context and evolution of dependency for older adults have been well delineated and supported in the literature as tied to the evolution of the welfare state. The problem can be viewed in terms of poverty and the policy response to poverty, which have either interrupted cycles of dependency for older adults or exacerbated their economic, health care, and health security needs (Berkman et al., 2006). The complexity of the dependency panorama for older adults and, specifically, elderly women, has not been sufficiently investigated. Elderly women are at higher risk for impoverishment and dependency than other older adults (Berkman et al., 2006). The relationship between dependency and suffering as social and public health problems cannot be ignored. The policy implications of this social and public health problem in the context of the findings of this study will be discussed below.

Socially Intelligible Maternal Care Facilities and Environments

In understanding the findings of both the research studies and the narratives, it is important to distinguish between the delivery system and its structures and processes, and praxes—the acts of agents (Laing & Esterson, 1970). The narratives of care facilities serving in a Maternal capacity for vulnerable elderly persons show that caregivers who are properly trained can provide the kind of relational, empathic Maternal care praxes that are being called for as part of the culture change movement, and that will make the person–Maternal–care–facility nexus "socially intelligible" (Laing & Esterson, 1970, p. 22). Shura and colleagues (2011) have turned to participatory action research in which the stakeholders themselves, such as the vulnerable residents, participate in research and help to investigate structure, process and change is responsive to elders' needs.

Palliative and End-of-Life Care Options in Long-Term Care

Access to adequate and appropriate care for seriously chronically ill persons is a major policy issue in the United States. In long-term care there are three principal care settings for persons approaching the end of life: care facilities, home care, and hospice care. Physicians and other health care professionals have not had conversations with persons about their end-of-life care wishes early enough or in enough depth, if they have had them at all. Csikai and Martin's (2010) study of referrals to hospice indicates that physicians do have conversations, but do not provide patients with enough information. Older adults are not having conversations with their health care professionals about their end-of-life wishes, and face major structural barriers to accessing appropriate care. Minority elders face particular barriers in accessing appropriate pain care in serious illness (IOM, 2011). Barriers encountered by seriously ill elderly persons need to be addressed from a systems perspective.

There has been groundbreaking progress in acknowledging the need for a national level focus on pain policy, and recognizing that it is an issue of global public health (Gostin, 2014). Pursuant to provisions of the Affordable Care Act, the IOM convened experts to study the problem and complexities of pain and, in 2011, released its "Relieving Pain in America: A Blueprint for Transforming Prevention, Care, Education, and Research." In follow-up to the IOM Report and Recommendation 2-2, the US Department of Health and Human Services established the NIH Interagency Pain Research Coordinating Committee. This committee is tasked with overseeing the development of a national strategy to improve pain care. As this national plan is developed, it will be important to examine current legal and regulatory frameworks as relevant to pain policy, especially access to an adequate and affordable supply of drugs.

Legal and Regulatory Framework for Drug Policy and Control

The framework of international treaties and federal and state regulations governing drug availability is complex and fragmented, especially when considering the type, scope, and limits of legal authority at each level. The Universal Declaration of Human Rights (1948); the United Nations' Single Convention on Narcotic Drugs of 1961, as amended by the 1972 Protocol Amending the Single Convention on Narcotic Drugs, 1961; the International Covenant on Economic, Social, and Cultural Rights (1966 [ICESR]); and the UN Committee on Economic, Social, and Cultural Rights, General Comment No. 14 (2000) have established the "right to the highest attainable standard of health" and its normative content, including rights to palliative care and relief from pain and suffering (Brennen, 2007; Connor & Sepulveda, 2014; Gilson, 2010; Joranson, Ryan, & Maurer, 2010). Inadequate treatment of pain or suffering may be a form of torture (Conner & Sepulveda, 2014). The Single Convention—a treaty to which the United States is a party—identifies "balance" as the overarching principle to guide policymaking that prevents drug diversion and abuse and provides adequate access to pain care through an available, accessible, and affordable drug supply (Gilson, 2010; Joranson, Ryan, & Maurer, 2010).

Federal government agencies—including the US Food and Drug Administration (FDA), the Drug Enforcement Administration, and the Centers for Disease Control and Prevention—play a large role in drug oversight and regulation. The Controlled Substances Act (1970 [CSA])—the major federal law governing controlled substances and narcotics—established a national system for classifying drugs and registering medication prescribers (Gilson, 2010). More recently, federal initiatives on pain have included two bills that establish new requirements on pain management for military personnel and veterans, as well as provisions of the National Pain Care Policy Act of 2009 (H.R. 756/S.660) that became part of the Affordable Care Act (2010) (Meghani et al., 2012). These provisions impose mandates that will advance pain care, research and education. At the administrative agency level, in July 2012 the FDA approved a Risk Evaluation and Mitigation Strategy (2012) for extended-release and long-acting opioids.

In light of states' legal authority to regulate the practice of health care, policymaking on pain and drug control has occurred mainly at the state level, with states serving as incubators of drug control policy. Almost all states have either established legal authority for, or already implemented, prescription drug monitoring programs to reduce the risk of drug diversion and opioid addiction. Researchers (Deyo et al., 2013; Perrone & Nelson, 2012) have reported wide variation among these programs in terms of design, function, access to data, and the monitored drugs, as well as sparse data measuring the programs' outcomes. These concerns highlight the need to focus on state pain policy implementation and evaluation, including states' palliative care laws and regulations.

Future Research

In 2011, the IOM developed a blueprint for pain research, and established workgroups under its Interagency Pain Research Coordinating Committee to develop more specific recommendations. One of the most important areas for future research is chronic pain—an experience not well understood. Chronic pain is a type of suffering and has certain qualities of unboundedness like suffering. Future research must explore the structure of chronic pain more and focus on understanding variation in pain and suffering experiences—especially across diverse and underserved populations and communities. Additional areas for investigation include comparative effectiveness, communication, pharmacological and non-pharmacological interventions (Reid et al., 2011), and the role of caregivers in influencing pain and suffering trajectories.

Practical Concerns in Ethical Sphere: Public Health, Phenomenology and Bioethics

The phenomenological lens on pain and suffering experience contributes to bioethical inquiry in ways that may be more fruitful than other ethical theories or approaches, especially principlism. Ethical theory in phenomenology concerns encounters with the other as subject; justification for ethical conduct which falls into the realm of normative ethics; and establishing the axiological grounds for ethical action that belongs in the domain of moral phenomenology.[2]

Ethical Encounter with the Other

Phenomenology's contribution to understanding the ethical encounter with the other as subject is perhaps its most unique and lasting contribution, and one that holds the greatest promise for breaking new ground in bioethics. Levinas (1969) makes a powerful case in phenomenology for an unmediated ethical encounter with the subject as other by recognizing the asymmetric moral claim of the other upon me. Levinas draws upon the Maternal as welcome and hospitality to describe this primal experience of intersubjectivity. Why is this view of the ethical encounter so novel?

The human person has to a large extent been viewed by natural science and to some extent by bioethics as inaccessible and as a suffering other in a private sphere. This private other is also thought to have a psychic life that is located only in the mind. Phenomenology turns this conceptualization of the private, inaccessible other with a mind closed in on itself upside down by demonstrating clearly, through accessing experience, that human beings are born into and live in a world of others whom they encounter in unmediated ways through pre-reflective and non-deductive processes of passive syntheses and empathy. Intersubjectivity as a ground for lived ethics and moral understanding is embedded in a larger historical and sociological movement in the human sciences that throws humankind—beyond solipsism, biomedical determinism, and wholly non-relational forms of autonomy and self-determination—toward fields of consciousness in which social contexts, social practices, and everyday as well as transcendent meanings are shared. This approach to grappling with ethical problems and conflicts has enormous possibilities for accessing unknown and unexplored worlds and horizons, and deepening understanding of fundamental humanity and meaning-making activity that reaches beyond the given possibility of strict appeal to ethical principles.

Levinas stands out as a phenomenologist who has asserted the primacy of ethics based on the presupposed and priority ethical claim of the other. He rejects modes of decision making that fail to recognize the irreducible otherness of each human being. However, Levinas avoids formal normative ethical theory in describing his version of ethics as pre-theoretical and pre-ontological.[3]

Normative Ethics and Relationship to Axiology

Husserl also bridged a long-standing divide between deontology and virtue ethics in the development of a normative ethics (Nenon, 2009). While Husserl integrates duty into his ethical perspective, he departs from Kant's idealism in articulating a relationship between subject and object in the constitution of consciousness, and in expanding the realm of reason to encompass feelings and evaluations in thetic position-taking. Unlike Kant, who saw no central place for inclinations in his formulation of duty and the categorical imperative, moral phenomenology clearly establishes the role of emotions in valuing. Husserl identifies doxic, axiological, and practical positions in intentional action. Position-taking and the synthesizing activity upon which empathy are based involve emotions, critical to a fundamental understanding of phenomenology and ethics.

Husserl grapples with the question of what constitutes a person and an ethical life. He introduces the concept of inner time consciousness, which integrates the past with the present and the future and forms the substrate of consciousness. For Husserl, this temporal process consists of evaluating one's beliefs, values, practical willingness, and character—and correcting them if they are not in consonance with one's motivations and desires. On one hand, Husserl identifies the intentional side of the subject as directed toward objective value structures in experience. On the other hand, he makes the role of free agency significant and recognized as an essential feature of living an authentically ethical life. Agency is inextricably tied to valuing and the role of emotions in valuing. Emotional responses to things found the value attributes the subject attaches to experience, and it is through this valuing that moral consciousness, moral goods, moral agency, and moral obligation and action arise (Drummond, 2008a).[4]

Application of Phenomenology to Selected Issues in Bioethics

While phenomenology has deep roots in philosophy, it is a practical science as much as a theoretical one. Husserl himself, as the father of phenomenology, is reportedly not known to have engaged in extensive practical applications of his theories and methods. However, today phenomenology is helping to bridge policy, research, and practice in such fields as psychiatry and community-based mental health. The introduction of the phenomenological attitude has transformed the delivery of mental health services and helped to reduce the stigma associated with mental health diagnoses. The application of phenomenology to experiences in health, illness, and decision making may have similar benefits for persons, families, caregivers, health professionals, and society. Narrative accounts of pain and suffering draw from phenomenological studies of these experiences.

Phenomenology calls into question conventional attitudes toward experience of consciousness that continue to torment bioethicists, such as dementia and autism. For example, typically, the person who develops dementia has a constituted empirical self that may be lost. The person, however, continues to live in the present—in a life-world that she/he is creating in the present moment. While memories of the old self may be memorialized by meaningful others and retained in the lived past and in social structures, the new self—the self with dementia—does not know oneself and is thrown into an unknown and unfamiliar everyday world with unknown others. What is this process of being newly worlded? It is at once a process of rupture and discontinuity, being dislocated from one's home and moorings, a trauma—and a rebirth that is a re-enactment of one's primordial beginnings. It is a process of discovery and locating one's agency that the new self navigates, albeit a different type of *relational* agency, moving between liminal states. What is preserved in these empirical changes, however, is what Husserl (1989) called the pure ego or the core immutable identity of a transcendental self. Scheler (1954) described this immutable identity that has no duration as personhood itself, a personhood that may be cut off from empirical moorings and is not subject to contingencies of empirical events.

Do things vary, by way of example, for persons who have had disabilities from birth, or are there essential features of personhood that are evident in the experience of autism? The subject with a disability, like the subject with dementia, is a subject in the present moment in a lived world with others. There are many parallels between persons with dementia and persons with disabilities in terms of retentions that may be memorialized by relational others and given continuity through social structures. Individuals with disabilities from birth are often perceived as lacking an originarily-given identity such as is given to one who develops dementia later in life. However, this is not correct: as even the person with a disability is born of a mother—and into intersubjectivity in the Maternal–fetal relationship—and experiences human development from its primordial beginnings. As such, and as Schütz writes, such a human person is not "concocted like homunculi in retorts," (Schutz, 1962, p. 168) but is a subject who is immediately present to and in simultaneous attunement with the other, sharing fluxes of time. In this "mutual tuning-in relationship," each person grasps and shares in the other's consciousness and makes a moral claim upon the other to be honored and treated with dignity.

Phenomenology establishes that both persons with dementia and persons with disabilities have originarily-given experience, are subjects and meaning-makers, and have a first-person perspective. Adoption of the third-person perspective of the natural sciences not only does not advance, but is destructive to, relational communication with persons who may appear to have bodies that are not like "mine" and with whom "I" may have difficulty making immediate assimilation. However, the grounds for empathy are abundant, in that persons with dementia and with any disability or impairment, by way of example, are human persons like "me" in many ways. They experience pain, they may see and hear, they have feelings, and they make the same moral claim as others do to honor them and treat them with dignity.

Phenomenology opens up new fields of fruitful inquiry in bioethics as it discloses the significance of the social world and the developmental origins of human experience. The phenomenological perspective helps illuminate the range and depth of moral experience in health and illness, as well as the limitations of medical science.[5]

Ethical Frameworks

In addressing ethical issues for seriously ill persons, we must clarify the frameworks in which we are situating our discussion. Clinical or practice ethics (Morrissey, 2014a) is helpful in locating the person in a dyadic relationship with her/his health care professionals. The focus of bioethical inquiry has historically focused on this relationship. However, a robust public health perspective on ethical issues has also emerged and been supported (Lee, 2012; Lee, Wright, & Semaan, 2013). The public health ethical perspective is focused on social relationship, but in the context of building community and solidarity. Phenomenology helps bridge the divide between clinical and public health ethics by giving us access to the social world in ordinary experience, and its origins. Instead of imposing pre-ordained or *a priori* principles of ethics from the outside, phenomenology fosters the development of free, moral agency and striving for the fulfillment of intentionalities through engagement with the world and with others. In phenomenology, it is understood that the world is already there and through our acts the world is disclosed and revealed to us. It is exactly this that is meant by grace (Rahner, 1967)—that which is given in the world. Several of the participants in the narratives spoke of grace in their testimony. Ethics in phenomenology is situated in an attitude of seeing the world, receiving its givens, and constituting the world in consciousness through the building up of experience.

Turning to the ethical problem of suffering, which I have seen and identified in the lived experience of seriously ill, elderly persons as losses of Maternal Foundations, passivity and receptivity, and a loss of intentional connection, an ethical response to suffering needs to be grounded in the conditions of possibility that will allow the suffering other to recover agency and attain the highest standards of health and well-being through human development. I have located that condition of possibility in a Maternal Ground, a given in our experience of the world in its otherness, and a gift of grace that is disclosed and revealed throughout the life course.

Strengthening Palliative Care Through Reflective Practice and Policy Advocacy

To strengthen palliative responses to suffering and the role of palliative care in improving care and quality of life for seriously ill elders, it becomes incumbent upon social workers and all helping professionals to engage in, practice and master the art of reflection from a stance of empathic attunement and immersion in elders' life-worlds. Phenomenology, which is a rigorous reflective methodology that is theoretical in its orientation, can inform and guide reflective practice (Schön, 1983). Schön's approach to reflection-in-action would situate health professionals and advocates in authentic life-world encounter with elderly persons and their intentionalities, fostering relational engagement, attitudes of mutual respect, as well as recognition of shared, reciprocal dignity and vulnerability (Benjamin, 2004). Soren Kierkegaard (1962) describes reflection as "the negation of immediacy" (p. 73). This positionality and attitude of "negating immediacy," even in a reflection-in-action mode of being, would bring a heightened awareness to bear on the strata of the relational moment with the elder who is suffering: i) the first-person experience of the suffering person who is a moral agent and decision maker; ii) the second-person perspective of the caregiver or advocate who stands in ethical relation to the person in pain, and in such capacity is called to provide embodied care and/or improve the conditions of possibility for such care; and iii) the multiple social, developmental, and relational contexts that form the ground of pain and suffering experience for the person, and create the care obligation to support the elder as a constituting agent in a movement toward hope and recovery in light of the elder's care needs, intentionalities, and strengths. In critically reflecting-on-action, that is, on the encounter with the elder after it has occurred, the social worker, health care practitioner or advocate opens up worldly engagements and contexts for questioning from a height that may help to inform interprofessional engagement and broad transdisciplinary collaboration in the service of improved health and well-being for seriously ill elders. Such height however is not meant to suggest that reflection involves abstraction from the concrete world. Rather, it is exactly the opposite—a focusing on being in the world in its full dimensionalities, negating the immediacy of the negation of non-being and emptiness, and solipsism in spatio-temporal existence, and restoring wholeness and interconnectedness through social relationship.

This multidimensional, layered, and dialectical process of reflection and feedback allows "dwelling" upon, "magnification, and amplification" (Wertz et al., 2011, p. 132) of the problem of knowledge in the fields of social work, psychology, nursing and medicine.

But the deeper processes of reflection are ones that do not necessarily concern knowledge building at all. Gabriel Marcel (1949) argues in *Being and Having* for reflection that goes beyond a primary layer of experience. He describes this process as a type of "reflection [that] will show us in the end that primary qualities are not necessarily endowed with an ontological priority over secondary qualities. Here again an intellectual hunger is at work..." (p. 140). Marcel powerfully suggests that this process of reflection is essentially spiritual in character.

Implications of Suffering Narratives

A highly rationalized, technocratic medical model of care can heighten suffering for the intended beneficiaries of medical care. Both the human dimensions of the suffering paradox and the limits of technical medical care are highlighted in the narratives. The palpable suffering of women and men afflicted with chronic pain and illness is compounded by often questionable surgeries, multiple rounds of radiation, or successive debridements—making the last months and days of their lives excruciatingly painful. Balancing the goals of person- and family-centered care with the goals of medicine, without adequately accounting for ethical compass, remains a struggle. Suffering is central to illness experience (Frank, 2001) and is deeply rooted in the human condition, yet cannot be ameliorated by uncapped investments in a medical model of care that puts a premium on technology.

The design and direction of our health systems, the education of our health professionals and pre-professional workforce, and the delivery of health care to persons and populations have missed the mark. While much has been written about issues which relate to questions of human suffering and ethical decision making such as access to hospice care (Jennings et al., 2003), there is a dearth of writing and research on the very question of human suffering itself—what suffering is, what it means, how it is assessed, and an ethical framework for understanding human agency in response to suffering. Turning to French Jewish philosopher Emmanuel Levinas, whose work in framing ethical responsibility to the other has been the basis of writing by Laurie Zoloth-Dorfman (1995), Ira Byock (2002) and Mark Freeman (2013), ethics in Levinas is made central to the relation between human beings and is the defining character of such relation (Levinas, 1969; 1981). As such, the ethical relation forms the ground of obligation for responsibility to the other. Levinasian ethics moves away from prescriptive moral theories and legislating ethical principles, and focuses instead on authentic human agency in responding to the call of the suffering other. Medical care—and the overarching social ecology of health and health decision making in which medicine is situated— must be informed by an understanding about accounting for the centrality of relationships and their ethical significance in health policy, clinical care and research. Whether diverse approaches to ethical questions in health care have been driven by a deontological, virtue ethics or relational perspective, the adoption of a starkly utilitarian calculus has historically decentered human relationships and human suffering. The detrimentality of this orientation calls for a radical shift in thinking and in allocation of resources.

There is some glimmer of change on the horizon. On both macro and micro levels, an unraveling at the margins of certain rigid frameworks in health care policy has begun. In the area of health decision making, challenges to the marginalization of the family and to the Western autonomy model have been advanced, and there is evidence of a movement toward shared decision-making models at both the bedside and at the systems levels (Brudney, 2009; Burt, 2005; Jennings & Morrissey, 2013; Morrissey & Jennings, 2006). There is growing evidence in support of the effectiveness of the national POLST (MOLST) paradigm in multiple care settings as a process model of decision making that brings persons, families, health care agents, surrogates and members of the health care team into conversation about the elder's goals of care (Bomba, Morrissey, & Leven, 2011; Sabatino & Karp, 2011). Promising work is also being done in the area of spiritual care that focuses on relationship, relatedness and meaning (Sulmasy, 2002; Puchalski et al., 2009; Puchalski et al., 2006; Doka, 2011). Daniel Sulmasy (2002) writes, "A human person is a being in relationship – biologically, psychologically, socially, and transcendentally. The patient is a human person. Illness disrupts all of the dimensions of relationship that constitute the patient as a human person..." (p. 32).

In looking toward the future, the critical question that emerges is how to carry out ethical responsibility to the other in diverse health care communities, ameliorate human suffering, and eliminate health and pain disparities (Meghani et al., 2012)—given our scarce resources. It is imperative in formulating health policy to reject a predominantly utilitarian calculus that fails to make human beings in relationship central to policy choices and decisions. Much of the research done to date shows that persons, and their families and caregivers, who are struggling with illness and suffering seek relational support and conversation. More vigorous and aggressive policy advocacy is needed in order to assure access to adequate structures for the provision of care including a better trained professional and pre-professional workforce across all fields in the health systems, and appropriate environmental provision, services and supports. Social workers, psychologists, nurses, chaplains, and generalist-level physicians and palliative care practitioners—who can spend time having conversations with persons and their families about the things that are important to them are essential to advancing goals of health and health reform. Reshaping a national agenda for health policy and research must start by prioritizing investments in human capital, not technology. The design of education and training programs for all health care practitioners will be critical to strengthening the workforce that serves frail elders struggling with serious illness and suffering. This education and training needs to be at the generalist level, and equip practitioners to perform basic pain assessments. Education should also focus on cultural sensitivity in serving individuals and groups with diverse backgrounds and experiences. It is in understanding human differences, family and cultural perspectives, experience of pain and suffering, and participation in shared decision-making processes with our loved ones that health professionals can provide the most appropriate integrated medical and social care to relieve the burdens of illness.

Final Thoughts and Reflections

I view my encounter with the suffering elders presented in the narratives as a gift of grace, as Karl Rahner has so well explained (1967), that cannot be properly accounted for within the conditions of human finitude. My access to suffering others, and the grace I received from each person as *other*, transcends yet at the same time is rooted in ordinary human experience and the common sense world. My most remarkable insight about these experiences and encounters is that there is always hope and possibility for attaining the highest forms of human development and well-being—even in the midst of the most abject and traumatic suffering.

Phenomenological studies of suffering may help to inform and guide professionals' and practitioners' work with seriously ill and suffering elders by facilitating recovery of a Maternal Ground for healing, agency, spiritual flourishing, resilience and hope. In addition, research studies and narratives such as these that provide portraits of human suffering experience may help influence policy makers to fashion broader palliative and social care provision to prevent and relieve suffering. The call to respond to the suffering other in the context of serious or life-limiting illness is first and foremost not an economic enterprise, but an essentially ethical one.

Notes

1　Morrissey, M. B. (2011). Expanding consciousness of suffering at the end of life: An ethical and gerontological response in palliative social work. Schützian Research, 3, 77–104. Zeta Books. Reproduced by permission.
2　Bioethics, 4E. © 2014 Gale, a part of Cengage Learning, Inc., p. 2396–2399. Reproduced by permission. www.cengage.com/permissions
3　Ibid., p. 2397.
4　Ibid., p. 2397.
5　Ibid., p. 2397–2399.

References

Ainsworth, M., & Bowlby, J. (1965). *Child care and the growth of love*. London: Penguin Books.

Altilio, T. (2004). Pain and symptom management: An essential role for social work. In J. Berzoff & P.R. Silverman (eds), Living with dying: Handbook for end-of-life healthcare practitioners (pp. 380-408). New York: Columbia University Press.

Atlas, S. J., & Skinner, J. (2010). Education and the prevalence of pain. In D. A. Wise (ed.), *Research findings in the economics of aging* (pp. 145–166). Chicago, IL: University of Chicago Press.

Bakan, D. (1968). Disease, pain & sacrifice: Toward a psychology of suffering. Beacon Press.

Bandura, A. (1977). *Social learning theory*. New Jersey: Prentice Hall.

——(1982). Self-efficacy mechanism in human agency. *American Psychologist*, *37*(20), 122–147.

——(1986). *Social foundations of thought and action: A social cognitive theory*. New Jersey: Prentice Hall.

Bandura, A. (1997). *Self-efficacy: The exercise of control*. New York: W.H. Freeman and Company.

Barber, M. D. (2010). Genetic phenomenology and potentiality: A new insight into the theory of empathy in Husserl. *Análisis: Revista Colombiana de Humanidades*, *75*, 61–89.

Barber, D. (2012). "The Cartesian Residue in Intersubjectivity and Child Development." *Schutzian Research* 4: 91–110.

Barber, M. (2011). *The intentional spectrum and intersubjectivity: Phenomenology and the Pittsburgh Neo-Hegelians*. Athens, OH: Ohio University Press.

Barber, M. D. (2013). *Alfred Schutz. Collected papers VI: Literary reality and relationships*. New York: Springer.

Barber, M. (2013). Alfred Schutz and the problem of empathy. In L. Embree and T. Nenon (eds), *Husserl's Ideen*. Dordrecht: Springer.

Barber, M. (2014). Resistance to pragmatic tendencies in the world of working in the religious finite province of meaning. Unpublished paper presented at Interdisciplinary Coalition of North American Phenomenologists, St. Louis.

Benjamin, J. (2004). Beyond doer and done: To an intersubjective view of thirdness. *Psychoanalytic Quarterly*, *73*(1), 5–46. doi:10.1200/JCO.2011.35.0561

Berkman, B., Gardner, D., Zodikoff, B., & Harootyan, L. (2006). Social work and aging in the emerging health care world. *Journal of Gerontological Social Work*, *48*(1/2), 203–217.

Black, H. (2006). Soul pain: The meaning of suffering in later life. Amityville, NY: Baywood Publishing Company, Inc.

Blacker, S., & Christ, G. (2011). Defining social work's role and leadership contributions in palliative care. In T. Altilio & S. Otis-Greene (eds), *Oxford textbook of palliative social work* (pp. 21–30). New York: Oxford University Press.

Bloom, P. (2013). *Just babies: Origins of good and evil*. New York: Crown Publishing Group, Random House.

Bomba, P., Morrissey, M. B., & Leven, D. C. (2011). Key role of social work in effective communication and conflict resolution process: Medical orders for life-sustaining treatment (MOLST) program in New York and shared medical decision making at the end of life. *Journal of Social Work in End-of-Life and Palliative Care*, *7*(1), 56–82.

Bowlby, J. (1957). An ethological approach to research in child development. *British Journal of Medical Psychology*, *30*, 230–240.

——(1958). The nature of the child's tie to his mother. *International Journal of Psycho-Analysis*, *39*, 350–373.

——(1960). Separation anxiety. *International Journal of Psycho-Analysis*, *41*, 69–113.

——(1965). *Child care and the growth of love* (2nd edn). London: Penguin.

——(1989). *Attachment and loss: Vol. 1: Attachment*. New York: Basic Books.

Brennen, F. (2007). Palliative care as an international human right. *Journal of Pain & Symptom Management 33*(5), 494–499.

Bretherton, I. (1992). The origins of attachment theory: John Bowlby and Mary Ainsworth. *Developmental Psychology*, *28*, 759–775.

Bronfenbrenner, U. (1979). *The ecology of human development*. Cambridge, MA: Harvard University Press.

Browning, D. (2004). Fragments of love: Explorations in the ethnography of suffering and professional caregiving. In J. Berzoff & P. R. Silverman (eds), *Living with dying: A handbook for end-of-life healthcare practitioners* (pp. 21–42). New York, NY: Columbia University Press.

Brudney, D. (2009). Choosing for another: Beyond autonomy and best interests. *Hastings Center Report*, *39*(2), 31–37.

Buber, M. (1958/2000). *I and Thou*. New York: Scribner.

Bugbee, H. (1958). *The inward morning: A philosophical exploration in journal form*. Athens, GA: University of Georgia Press.

Burlea, S. R. (2009). Encountering the suffering other in illness narratives: Between the Memory of suffering and the suffering memory. Unpublished dissertation. Montreal University.

Burt, R. (2005). The end of autonomy. In B. Jennings, G. Kaebnick & T. H. Murray (eds), *Improving end of life care: Why has it been so difficult? Hastings Center Report Special Supplement*, 35(6), S9–S13.

Byock, I. (1996). The nature of suffering and the nature of opportunity at the end-of-life. *Clinics of Geriatric Medicine*, *12*, 237–251.

——(1997). *Dying well: Peace and possibilities at the end of life*. New York: Riverhead Books.

——(2002). The meaning and value of death. *Journal of Palliative Medicine*, *5*(2), 279–288.

Cacioppo, J., & Patrick, W. (2008). *Loneliness: Human nature and need for social connection*. W. W. Norton & Company.

Cagle, J. G., & Altilio, T. (2011). The social work role in pain and symptom management. In T. Altilio & S. Otis-Green (eds), *Oxford textbook of palliative social work* (pp. 271–286). New York: Oxford University Press.

Callahan, D. (2011). Rationing: theory, politics, and passions. *Hastings Center Report, 41*(2), 23–27.

Cassell, E. J. (1982). The nature of suffering and the goals of medicine. *New England Journal of Medicine, 306,* 639–645.

——(1999). Diagnosing suffering: A perspective. *Annals of Internal Medicine, 131*(7), 531–534.

——(2004). *Nature of suffering and the goals of medicine* (2nd edn). New York: Oxford University Press.

Charmaz, K. (1983). Loss of self: A fundamental form of suffering in chronically ill. *Sociology of Health and Illness, 5*(2), 168–195.

——(1997). *Good days, bad days: The self in chronic illness and time*. New Brunswick, New Jersey: Rutgers University Press.

——(1999). Stories of suffering: Subjective tales and research narratives. *Qualitative Health Research,* 9(3), 362–382.

Churchill, S. (2010). "Second person" perspectivity in observing and understanding emotional expression. In L. Embree, M. Barber & T. J. Nenon (eds), *Phenomenology 2010. Volume 5: Selected essays from North America. Part 2: Phenomenology beyond philosophy,* (pp. 23–104). Bucharest: Zeta Books/Paris: Arghos-Diffusion.

Connor, S., & Sepulveda, C. M. (eds) (2014). *Global atlas of palliative care at the end of life*. Geneva/London: World Health Organization and Worldwide Palliative Care Alliance.

Cox, C. (2005). *Community care for an aging society: Issues, policies and services*. New York: Springer Publishing Company.

Csikai, E. L., & Martin, S. S. (2010). Bereaved hospice caregivers' views of the transition to hospice. *Social Work in Health Care,* 49, 387–400.

Davidson, L. (2003). *Living outside mental illness: Qualitative studies of recovery in schizophrenia.* New York: New York University Press.

Davidson, L., & Cosgrove, L. (2002). Psychologism and phenomenological psychology revisited, Part II: The return to positivism. *Journal of Phenomenological Psychology,* 33, 2.

De Beauvoir, S. (1965). *A very easy death.* New York: Pantheon Books.

Dekkers, W. (2001). Coming home. On the goals of palliative care. In H. ten Have & R. Janssens, *Palliative care in Europe* (pp. 117–126). Netherlands: IOS Press.

DeRobertis, E. M. (2010). Winnicott, Kohut, and the developmental context of well-being. *The Humanistic Psychologist, 38*(4), 336–354.

Deyo, R. A., Irvine, J. M., Millet, L. M., Beran, T., O'Kane, N., Wright, D. A., & McCarty, D. (2013). Measures such as interstate cooperation would improve the efficacy of programs to track controlled drug prescriptions. *Health Affairs, 32*(3), 1–11.

Doka, K. J. (2011). Religion and spirituality: Assessment and intervention. *Journal of Social Work in End-of-Life Palliative Care, 7*(1), 99–109.

Drummond, J. J. (2002). Aristotelianism and Phenomenology. In J. J. Drummond & Lester E. Embree, *Phenomenological Approaches to Moral Philosophy: A Handbook* (pp. 15–46). Netherlands: Kluwer Academic Publishers.

———(2008a). Moral phenomenology and moral intentionality. *Phenomenology and the Cognitive Sciences*, 7(1), 35–49.

———(2008b). *Historical dictionary of Husserl's philosophy*. Maryland: Scarecrow Press, Inc.

Dumm, T. (2008). *Loneliness as a way of life*. Cambridge, MA: Harvard University Press.

Embree, L. (1997). What is phenomenology? In L. Embree, E. A. Behnke, D. Carr, J. C. Evans, J. Huertas-Jourda, J. J. Kockelmans & R. M. Zaner (eds), *Encyclopedia of phenomenology* (Vol. 18, pp. 1–10). Boston, MA: Kluwer Academic.

———(2010a). Interdisciplinarity within phenomenology. *Indo-Pacific Journal of Phenomenology*, *10*, 1–6. (Appeared October 2010 in Castilian as La Interdisciplinaridad dentro de la Fenomenología. *Investigaciones Fenomenológicas*, *8*, 9–22.)

———(2010b). Founding some practical disciplines in Schützian social psychology. *Bulletin d'analyse phénoménologique*, 6. Available at: http://popups.ulg.ac.be/1782-2041/index. php?id=370 (accessed June 10, 2013).

———(2003). The possibility of constitutive phenomenology of the environment. In C. S. Brown & T. Toadvine (eds), Eco-Phenomenology: Back to the Earth itself (pp. 37–50). New York: State University of New York Press.

Emirbayer, M., & Mische, A. (1998). What is agency? *American Journal of Sociology*, *103*(4), 962–1023.

Erikson, E. H. (1950/1963). *Childhood and society*. New York: Norton.

———(1959/1980). *Identity and the life cycle*. New York: Norton.

Estes, C. L. (2001). *Social policy and aging: A critical perspective*. Thousand Oaks: Sage Publications.

Ferrell, B., & Coyle, N. (2008). *The nature of suffering and the goals of nursing*. New York: Oxford University Press.

Fins, J. J. (2006). *A palliative ethic of care: Clinical wisdom at life's end*. Sudbury, MA: Jones and Bartlett.

Foucault, M. (1995). *Discipline and punishment*. New York: Vintage Books.

Frank, A. W. (1978). Anxiety aroused by the dying: A phenomenological inquiry. *Journal of Phenomenological Psychology*, *9*(1), 99–113.

———(1995). *The wounded storyteller*. Chicago: University of Chicago Press.

———(2001). Can we research suffering? *Qualitative Health Research*, *11*(3), 353–362.

Frankl, V. E. (1984). *Man's search for meaning*. Boston, MA: Beacon Press.

Freeman, M. (2008a). Beyond narrative: Dementia's tragic promise. In L. C. Hyden & J. Brockmeier (eds), *Health, illness and culture* (pp. 169–184). New York: Routledge.

———(2008b). Life without narrative? Autobiography, dementia, and the nature of the real. In G. O. Mazur (ed.), *Thirty year commemoration to the life of A.R. Luria* (pp. 129–144). New York: Semenko Foundation.

———(2013). *Priority of the other: Thinking and living beyond the self*. New York: Oxford University Press.

Freud, A. (1948). The psychoanalytic study of infantile feeding disturbances. *Psychoanalytic Study of the Child*, *2*, 119–132.

———(1952). The mutual influence in the development of ego. *Psychoanalytic Study of the Child*, *7*, 42–50.

———(1954). Psychoanalysis and education. *Psychoanalytic Study of the Child*, *9*, 9–15.

———(1965). *Normality and pathology in childhood: Assessments of development*. New York: International Universities Press.

Freud, S. (1930). *Civilization and its discontents*. New York: Norton, 1986.

——(1953). The "uncanny". An infantile neurosis and other works. In J. Strachey (ed. and trans.) *The standard edition of the complete psychological works of Sigmund Freud, Volume XVII (1917–1919)*, pp. 217–256. London: Hogarth Press.

Gallagher, S. (2007). The natural philosophy of agency. *Philosophy Compass, 2*, 347–357.

Garbarino, J. (1999). *Lost boys: Why our sons turn violent and how we can save them.* New York: Free Press.

Gatchel, R. J., McGreary, D. D., McGreary, C. A., & Lippe, B. (2014). Interdisciplinary pain management: Past, present and future. *American Psychologist, 69* (2), 119–130.

Geniusas, S. (2010). What does the question of origins mean in phenomenology? In M. Barber, L. Embree, & J. Nenon (eds), *Phenomenology 2010: Selected Essays from North America, Part I, Phenomenology within Philosophy* (pp. 81–94). Bucharest: Zeta Books.

Gibson, James J. (1979). *The ecological approach to visual perception.* New Jersey, USA: Lawrence Erlbaum Associates.

Gilligan, C. (1993). *In a different voice.* Mass: Harvard University Press.

Gilson, A. M. (2010). Laws and policies involving pain management. In J. C. Ballantyne, J. P. Rathmell, & S. M. Fishman (eds), *Bonica's management of pain* (4th edn) (pp. 166–182). Philadelphia, PA: Lippincott, Williams & Wilkins.

Giorgi, A. (1970). *Psychology as a human science.* New York: Harper & Row.

——(2009). *The descriptive phenomenological method in psychology: A modified Husserlian approach.* Pittsburgh, PA: Duquesne University Press.

Goffman, E. (1961). *Asylums: Essays on the social situation of mental patients and other inmates.* New York: Anchor Books.

Gomez-Baptiste, X., Martinez-Munoz, M., Blay, C., Espinosa, J., Contel, J. C. & Ledesma, A. (2012). Identifying needs and improving palliative care of chronically ill patients: a community-oriented, population-based, public-health approach. Curr Opin Support Palliat Care. 6(3):371–8. doi: 10.1097/SPC.0b013e328356aaed

Gonzalez Sanders, D. J., & Fortinsky, R. H. (2012). *Dementia care with Black and Latino Families. A social work problem-solving approach.* New York: Springer Publishing Company.

Good, B. J. (1994). The body, illness experience, and the lifeworld: A phenomenological account of chronic pain. In Byron J. Good (ed.), *Medicine, Rationality and Experience: An anthropological perspective* (pp. 116–134). Cambridge: Cambridge UP.

Gostin, L. (2014). *Global health law.* Boston, MA: Harvard University Press.

Greene, R. R., & Cohen, H. L. (2005). Social work with older adults and their families: Changing practice paradigms. *Families in Society, 86*(3), 367–373.

Guntrip, H. (1985). *Psychoanalytic theory, therapy and the self.* London: Karnac Books.

Gwyther, L. P., Altilio, T., Blacker, S., Christ, G., Csikai, E. L., Hooyman, N., Kramer, B, & Howe, J. (2005). Social work scope of practice and competencies essential to palliative care, end-of-life care, and grief work. *Journal of Social Work in End-of-Life and Palliative Care, 1*(1), 87–120.

Hamington, M. (2004). *Embodied care: Jane Addams, Maurice Merleau-Ponty, and feminist ethics.* Chicago: University of Illinois Press.

Hawkley, L. C., Hughes, M. E., Waite, L. J., Masi, C. M., Thisted, R. A., & Cacioppo, J. T. (2008). From social structural factors to perceptions of relationship quality and loneliness: The Chicago health, aging and social relations study. *J Gerontol B Psychol Sci Soc Sci., 63B*(6), S375–S384.

Higgins, P. C. (2011). Guess who's coming to dinner? The emerging identity of palliative social workers. In T. Altilio & S. Otis-Greene (eds), *Oxford textbook of palliative social work*, (pp. 31–42). New York: Oxford University Press.

Hooyman, N. R., & Kramer, B. J. (2006). *Living through loss: Interventions across the lifespan.* New York: Columbia University Press.

Husserl, E. (1900–01/1970). *Logical investigations* (J. N. Findlay, Trans.). London: Routledge & Kegan Paul Ltd.

——(1954/1970). The crisis of European sciences and transcendental phenomenology: An introduction to phenomenological philosophy. (D. Carr, Trans.) Evanston: Northwestern University Press.

——(1913/1982). *Ideas pertaining to a pure phenomenology and to a phenomenological philosophy. First book: General introduction to a pure phenomenology* (F. Kersten, Trans.). The Hague: Martinus Nijhoff Publishers.

——(1913/1989). *Ideas pertaining to a pure phenomenology and to a phenomenological philosophy. Second book: Studies in the phenomenology of constitution* (R. Rojcewicz & A. Schuwer, Trans.). Dordrecht, The Netherlands: Kluwer Academic Publishers.

——(1948/1973). *Experience and judgment: Investigations in a genealogy of logic* (L. Landgrebe, ed.; J. S. Churchill & K. Ameriks, Trans.). Evanston, IL: Northwestern University Press.

——(1962/1977). *Phenomenological psychology: Lectures, summer semester, 1925* (Q. Scanlon, Trans.). Boston: Martinus Nijhoff Publishers.

Institute of Medicine. (2011). *Relieving pain in America: A blueprint for transforming prevention, care, education, and research.* Washington DC: National Academies Press.

International Association for the Study of Pain (IASP). (2011). *IASP taxonomy.* Available at: www.iasp-pain.org/AM/Template.cfm?Section=Pain_Defi..isplay.cfm&ContentID= 1728 (accessed April 17, 2011)

Jager, B. (1979). Dionysos and the world of passion. In A. Giorgi, R. Knowles, & D. L. Smith, *Duquesne Studies in Phenomenological Psychology, Vol. III* (pp. 209–226). Pittsburgh: Duquesne University Press.

Jager, B. (1999). Eating as natural event and as intersubjective phenomenon: Toward a Phenomenology of Eating. *Journal of Phenomenological Psychology*, 30(1), 66–116.

Jennings, B. (2007). Public health and civic republicanism: Toward an alternative framework for public health ethics. In A. Dawson, & M. Verweij (eds), *Ethics, prevention, and public health* (pp. 30–58). Oxford: Oxford University Press.

——(2009). Agency and moral relationship in dementia. *Metaphilosophy*, 40, 425–437.

Jennings, B., & Morrissey, M. B. (2013). Health care costs in end of life and palliative care: the quest for ethical reform. In M.B. Morrissey & B. Jennings (Eds.), Partners in Palliative Care: Enhancing Ethics in Care at the End-of-Life, (pp. 109–126). New York: Routledge.

Jennings, B., Ryndes, T., D'Onofrio, C., & Baily, M. A. (2003). Access to hospice care: Expanding boundaries, overcoming barriers. *Hasting Center Report Special Supplement, 33*(2), S3–S7.

Jensen, M. P., & Turk, D. C. (2014). Contributions of psychology to the understanding and treatment of people with chronic pain: Why it matters to all psychologists. *American Psychologist, 69*(2), 105–118.

Joranson, D. E., Ryan, K. M., & Maurer, M. A. (2010). Disparities in opioid policy, availability, and access: The way forward. In J. C. Ballantyne, J. P. Rathmell, & S. M. Fishman, (eds), *Bonica's management of pain* (pp. 194–208). Philadelphia, PA: Lippincott, Williams & Wilkins.

Josselson, R. (2013). Interviewing for Qualitative Inquiry: A relational approach. New York: Guilford Press.

Kamens, S. R., Forgione, F., Minahan, J., & Driggs, I. (2014, March). Anomalous and psychotic experiences in total institutions: Experiences of inpatients in an urban psychiatric hospital. Unpublished paper presentation at the Society for Humanistic Psychology annual conference, Palo Alto, California.

Karantzas, G. C., Evans, L., & Foddy, M. (2010). The role of attachment in current and future parent caregiving. J Gerontol B Psychol Sci Soc Sci., *65*(5), 573–580.

Kierkegaard, S. (1962). *The point of view for my work as an author*. Edited by Benjamin Nelson. New York: Harper & Row Publishers, Inc.

Kleinman, A. (1988). *The illness narratives.* New York: Basic Books.

——(2012). The art of medicine: Caregiving as moral experience. *The Lancet, 380* (9853), 1550–1551.

Kleinman, A., & Kleinman, J. (1997). The appeal of experience, the dismay of images: Cultural appropriations of suffering in our times. In A. Kleinman, V. Das, & M. Lock (eds), *Social suffering* (pp. 1–24). Los Angeles, CA: University of California Press.

Labouvie-Vief (1999). Emotions in adulthood. In V. L. Bengtson, & K. Warner Schaie (eds), *Handbook of Theories of Aging*, (pp. 253–267). New York: Springer Publishing Company, Inc.

LaCoursiere, R. B. (2010). Impact of Arts participation on health outcomes of older adults… Dying calls for mother – factual or fanciful? *Journal of Aging, Humanities and Arts*, 4 (4), 415–410.

Laing, R. D., & Esterson, A. (1970). *Sanity, madness & the family.* New York: Penguin.

Lee, L. (2012). Public health ethics Theory: Review and path to convergence. *Journal of Law, Medicine & Ethics*, 34(1), 85–98.

Lee, L., Wright, B., & Semaan, S. (2013). Expected ethical competencies of public health professionals and graduate curricula in accredited schools of public health in North America. *American Journal of Public Health*, *103*(5), 938–942.

Levinas, E. (1969). *Totality and infinity: An essay on exteriority.* Pittsburgh, PA: Duquesne University Press.

——(1981). *Otherwise than being or beyond essence.* Pittsburgh, PA: Duquesne University Press.

Lunney, J. R., Lynn, J., & Hogan, C. (2002). Profiles of older Medicare decedents. *Journal of the American Geriatrics Society*, 50, 1108–1112.

Lynn, J. (2005). Living long in fragile health: The new demographics shape end of life care. In B. Jennings, G. Kaebnick, & T. Murray (eds), *Improving end of life care: why has it been so difficult? Hastings Center Report Special Report*, *35*(6), S14–S18.

McGrenere, J., & Ho, W. (2000). Affordances: Clarifying and evolving a concept. In Proceedings of Graphics Interface 2000, May 15–17, 2000, Montreal, Quebec, Canada, pp. 179–186.

Marcel, G. (1949). *Being and having* (K. Farrer, Trans.). Westminster, London: Dacre Press.

——(1962). *Homo Viator: Introduction to a metaphysic of hope.* New York: Harper Torchbooks.

——(1964). *Creative fidelity*, Translated, with an introduction, by R. Rosthal. New York: Farrar, Strauss & Company.

Maslow, H. (1954) *Motivation and personality* (3rd edn). New York: HarperCollins.

Maxwell, J. A. (2005). *Qualitative research design: An interactive approach* (2nd edn). Thousand Oaks, CA: Sage Publications.

Meghani, S. H., Polomano, R. C., Tait, R. C., Vallerand, A. H., Anderson, K. O., & Gallagher, R. M. (2012). Advancing a national agenda to eliminate disparities in pain care: Directions for health policy, education, practice, and research. *Pain Medicine*, *13*(1), 5–28.

Merleau-Ponty, M. (1945/1962). *Phenomenology of perception* (C. Smith, Trans.). London: Routledge & Kegan Paul.

——(1964). *The primacy of perception and other essays on phenomenological psychology, the philosophy of art, history and politics* (J. M. Edie, ed.; W. Cobb, trans.). Evanston, IL: Northwestern University Press.

——(1964). *The child's relations with others* (W. Cobb, trans.). In J. M. Edie (ed.), *The primacy of perception*. Evanston, IL: Northwestern University Press.

Merton, T. (1966). *Raids on the Unspeakable*. New York: New Directions Publishing Co.

Meyer, C. (1983). The search for coherence. In C. Meyer (ed.), *Clinical social work in the ecosystems perspective* (pp. 5–34). New York: Columbia University Press.

Miller, R. B. (2004). *Facing human suffering: Psychology and psychotherapy as moral engagement.* Washington, DC: American Psychological Association.

Miller, S. C., Mor, V., Wu, N., Gozalo, P., & Lapan, K. (2002). Does receipt of hospice care in nursing homes improve the management of pain at the end of life? *Journal of American Geriatrics Society*, 50, 507–515.

Mor, V., Zinn, J., Angelelli, J., Teno, J. M., & Miller, S. C. (2004). Driven to tiers: Socioeconomic and racial disparities in the quality of nursing home care. *Millbank Quarterly*, 82, 227–256.

Morrissey, M. B. (1979). Virginia Woolf: The affirmation of life in the being-in-spirit. Unpublished thesis manuscript. Fordham University.

——(2011a). Phenomenology of pain and suffering: A humanistic perspective in gerontological health and social work. *Journal of Social Work in End-of-Life and Palliative Care*, *7*(1), 14–38.

——(2011b). Suffering and decision making among seriously ill elderly women. Unpublished Dissertation, Fordham University.

——(2011c). Expanding consciousness of suffering at the end of life: An ethical and gerontological response in palliative social work. Schützian Research, Special Issue: *Phenomenology of the Human Sciences*, *3*, 79–106.

——(2014a). Ethical issues. *Cultural Sociology of Mental Illness: An A-to-Z Guide* (pp. 282–288). Andrew Scull (ed.), Thousand Oaks, CA: Sage.

——(2014b). Merleau-Ponty. Maurice. *Cultural Sociology of Mental Illness: An A-to-Z Guide* (pp. 530–531). Andrew Scull (ed.), Thousand Oaks, CA: Sage.

——(2014c). Patient accounts of illness. *Cultural Sociology of Mental Illness: An A- to-Z Guide*. Andrew Scull (ed.), Thousand Oaks, CA: Sage.

Morrissey, M. B., & Barber, M. (2014). Phenomenology. *Bioethics*, 4th edn. (2014). Edited by Bruce Jennings. Farmington Hills, MI: Macmillan Reference USA.

Morrissey, M. B., & Jennings, B. (2006). A social ecology of health model in end-of-life decision-making: Is the law therapeutic? *New York State Bar Association. Health Law Journal. Special Edition: Selected Topics in Long-Term Care Law*, *11*(1), 51–60.

Morrissey, M. B., Viola, D., & Shi, Q. (2014). Relationship between pain and chronic illness among seriously ill older adults: Expanding role for palliative social work. *Journal of Social Work in End-of-Life and Palliative Care*, *10*(1), 8–33.

National Association of Social Workers. (2004). *Standards for social work practice in palliative and end of life care*. Washington, DC: NASW Press.

——(2008). *Code of ethics*. Washington, DC: NASW Press.

National Consensus Project (2013). *Clinical practice guidelines for quality palliative Care*, 3rd edn. Available from: www.nationalconsensusproject.org/GuidelinesTOC.pdf (accessed November 30, 2013).

Nelson-Becker, H. B. (2006). Voices of resilience: Older adults in hospice care. *Journal of Social Work in End of Life & Palliative Care*, *2*(3), 87–106.

Nenon, Thomas J. (2011). Reason and feeling in Husserl's later lectures on ethics (in Japanese translation). *Tetsugaku-Zasshi (Journal of Philosophy)* 76: 147–170.

Neuman, K. (2013). More usable Winnicott. *Psychoanalytic Inquiry*, *33*(1), 59–68.

Nussbaum, M. C. (2001). *Upheavals of thought: The intelligence of emotions*. New York: Cambridge University Press.

O'Brien, M. B. (2011). Practical necessity: A study in ethics, law, and human action. University of Texas Libraries. Available at: http://repositories.lib.utexas.edu/handle/2152/ETD-UT-2011-05-3257 (accessed August 27, 2013).

Orange, D. (2011). *The suffering stranger*. New York: Routledge.

Padgett, D. K. (2008). *Qualitative methods in social work research*. Thousand Oaks, CA: Sage Publications, Inc.

Palos, G. R. (2011). Social work research agenda in palliative and end-of-life care. In T. Altilio & S. Otis-Greene (eds), *Oxford textbook of palliative social work*, (pp. 719–733). New York: Oxford University Press.

Parsonnet, L., & Lethoborg, C. (2011). Addressing suffering in end of life care: Two psychotherapeutic models. In T. Altilio & S. Otis-Greene (eds), *Oxford textbook of palliative social work*. New York: Oxford University Press.

Patton, M. Q. (2002). *Qualitative research and evaluation methods* (3rd edn). Thousand Oaks, CA: Sage Publications, Inc.

Perrone, J., & Nelson, L. (2012). Medication reconciliation for controlled substances—An "ideal" prescription-drug monitoring program. *New England Journal of Medicine*, *366*, 2341–2343. doi:10.1056/NEJMp1204493

Piaget, J. (1932). *The moral judgment of the child*. Glencoe, IL: Free Press.

Picasso, P. (1903–04). *The Old Guitarist*. [Painting.] Available at: www.artic.edu/aic/collections/artwork/28067 (accessed December 15, 2013).

——(1937). *Guernica*. [Painting.] Available at: www.museoreinasofia.es/coleccion/obra/guernica (accessed December 15, 2013).

Puchalski, C., Ferrell, B., Virani, R., et al. (2009). Improving the quality of spiritual care as a dimension of palliative care: The report of the consensus conference. *Journal of Palliative Medicine*, *12*(10), 885–903.

Puchalski, C. M., Lunsford, B., Harris, M. H., & Miller, R. T. (2006). Interdisciplinary spiritual care for seriously ill and dying patients: A collaborative model. *Cancer Journal*, 12(5), 398–416.

Rahner, K. *Theological Investigations*, 20 vols. New York: Crossroad, 1961–83.

Rahner, K. Reflections on the Experience of Grace. *Theological Investigations III*, trans. Karl H. and Boniface Kruger, OFM (Baltimore, MD: Helicon Press, 1967; originally published by Einsiedeln, Benziger in 1956 as Zur Theologie des geistlichen Lebens), 87–88.

Reid, C. et al. (2011). Improving the pharmacologic management of pain in older adults: Identifying the research gaps and methods to address them. *Pain Medicine*, *12*, 1336–1357.

Reinhard, S. C., Levine, C., & Samis, S. (2012). *Home alone: Family caregivers providing complex chronic care*. Washington, DC: AARP Public Policy Institute.

——(2014). Family caregivers providing complex chronic care to their spouses. Washington, DC: AARP Public Policy Institute.

Roberts, M. J., & Reich, M. R. (2002). Ethical analysis in public health. *The Lancet, 359,* no. 9311, 1055–1059.

Roche, M. W. (2005). The greatness and limits of Hegel's theory of tragedy. *A Companion to Tragedy.* Ed. Rebecca Bushnell (pp. 51–67). Oxford: Blackwell.

Rogers, C. R. (1961). *On becoming a person.* Boston: Houghton-Mifflin.

Rogers, M. (2008). Constituted to care: Alfred Schütz and the feminist ethic of care. Unpublished paper. Ramapo College, New Jersey.

Ryan, K., Todres, L., & Alexander, J. (2010). The calling, permission and fulfillment: The interembodied experience of suffering. *Qualitative Health Research,* 1–12.

Sabatino, C., & Karp, N. (2011). Improving advanced illness care: The evolution of state POLST programs. Washington, DC: AARP Public Policy Institute.

Sass, L., Parnas, J., & Zahavi, D. (2011). Phenomenological psychopathology and schizophrenia: Contemporary approaches and misunderstandings. *Philosophy, Psychiatry, & Psychology, 18*(1), 1–23.

Saunders, D. C. (2011). Social work and palliative care – The early history. In T. Altilio & S. Otis-Green (eds), *Oxford textbook of palliative social work* (pp. 5–10). New York: Oxford University Press.

Scheler, M. (1954). *The nature of sympathy.* New Haven: Yale University Press.

Schön, D. (1983). *The reflective practitioner: How professionals think in action.* New York: Basic Books.

Schütz, A. (1942/1962). Scheler's theory of intersubjectivity and the general thesis of the alter ego. In M. Natanson (ed.), *Collected papers I.* The Hague: Martinus Nijhoff Publishers.

——(1943/1964). The problem of rationality in the social world. In A. Broderson (ed.), *Collected papers II.* The Hague: Martinus Nijhoff Publishers.

——(1944). The Stranger: An essay in social psychology. *American Journal of Sociology, 49* (6), 499–507.

——(1951). Making music together—A study in social relationship. *Social Research, 18*(1/4), 76.

——(1957/1966). The problem of transcendental intersubjectivity in Husserl. In I. Schütz (ed.), *Collected papers III.* The Hague: Martinus Nijhoff Publishers.

——(1967). *The phenomenology of the social world,* G. Walsh & F. Lehnert (trans.). Evanston, IL: Northwestern University Press.

——(1962/1973). *Collected papers: The problem of social reality,* 4th edn, M. Natanson (ed.). The Hague: Martinus Nijhoff Publishers.

——(1996). *Collected papers IV,* H. Wagner (ed.). The Hague: Martinus Nijhoff Publishers.

Shura, R., Siders, R., & Dannefer, D. (2011). Culture change in long-term care: Participatory action research and the role of the resident. *Gerontologist, 51*(2), 212–225.

Simms, E.-M. (2001). Milk and flesh: A phenomenological reflection on infancy and coexistence. *Journal of Phenomenological Psychology, 32*(1), 22–40.

Slochower, J. (2014). *Holding and psychoanalysis: A relational perspective.* NY: Routledge.

Stapleton, T. J. (1983). *Husserl and Heidegger: The question of a phenomenological beginning.* Albany: State University of New York Press.

Starr, K. (2008). *Repair of the soul: Metaphors of transformation in Jewish mysticism and psychoanalysis.* New York: Routledge.

Stern, D. (1985). *The interpersonal world of the infant: A view from psychoanalysis and developmental psychology.* New York: Basic Books.

Stjernswärd, J., Foley, K. M., & Ferris, F. D. (2007). The public health strategy for palliative care. *Journal of Pain and Symptom Management, 33*(5), 486–493.

Stone, D. A., & Papadimitriou, C. (2011). Exploring Heidegger's ecstatic temporality in the context of embodied breakdown. Schützian Research, 2/2010, 136–152.

Sulmasy, D. P. (2002). A biopsychosocial-spiritual model for the care of patients at the end of life. *Gerontologist, 42,* 24–33.

Summers, F. (2013). *The psychoanalytic vision: The experiencing subject, transcendence, and the therapeutic process.* New York: Routledge.

Takahashi, K. (2005). Toward a life-span theory of close relationships: The affective relationships model. In M. Lewis & K. Takahashi (eds), *Beyond the dyad: Conceptualization of social networks.* Switzerland: Karger Publishers.

United Nations. (1948). *Universal Declaration of Human Rights*, 10 December 1948, 217 A (III). Available at: www.un.org/en/documents/udhr/ (accessed January 26, 2014).

United Nations. (1977). Single Convention on Narcotic Drugs, 1961, as amended by the 1972 Protocol Amending the Single Convention on Narcotic Drugs, 1961. New York: United Nations, 1977. Available at: https://treaties.un.org/Pages/ShowMTDSGDetails. aspx?src=UNTSONLINE&tabid=2&mtdsg_no=VI-17&chapter=6&lang=en#Particip ants (accessed January 26, 2014).

——(1996). *International Covenant on Economic, Social and Cultural Rights*, 16 December 1966, United Nations, Treaty Series, vol. 993, p. 3. Available at: https:// treaties.un.org/Pages/ViewDetails.aspx?mtdsg_no=IV-3&chapter=4&lang=en (accessed January 26, 2014).

——(2000). Committee on Economic, Social and Cultural Rights (CESCR), *General Comment No. 14: The Right to the Highest Attainable Standard of Health (Art. 12 of the Covenant)*, 11 August 2000, E/C.12/2000/4. Available at: www.un.org/documents/ ecosoc/docs/2001/e2001-22.pdf (accessed January 26, 2014).

Warner, E., & Gualtiere-Reed, T. (2014). Improving care for people with serious illness through innovative payer-provider partnerships. A palliative care toolkit and resource guide. New York: Center to Advance Palliative Care.

Webb, N. B. (2011). *Social work practice with children.* New York: Guilford Press.

Weiss, G. (2008). *Refiguring the ordinary.* Indianapolis: Indiana University Press.

Wertz, F. J. (1981). The birth of the infant: A developmental perspective. *Journal of Phenomenological Psychology, 12*(1), 205–220.

——(1983a). From everyday to psychological description: Analyzing the moments of a qualitative data analysis. *Journal of Phenomenological Psychology, 14*(2), 197–241.

——(1983b). Some constituents of descriptive psychological reflection. *Human Studies, 6*(1), 35–51.

——(1985). Methods and findings in an empirical analysis of "being criminally victimized." In A. Giorgi (ed.), *Phenomenology and psychological research* (pp. 155–216). Pittsburgh, PA: Duquesne University Press.

——(2005). Phenomenological research methods for counseling psychology. *Journal of Counseling Psychology, 52*(2), 167–177.

——(2008). The role of the humanistic movement in the history of psychology. *Journal of Humanistic Psychology,* 48, 221–242.

——(2010). The method of eidetic analysis for psychology. In T. Cloonan & C. Thiboutot (eds), *The redirection of psychology: Essays in honor of Amedeo P. Giorgi*, pp. 261–278).

Montreal, Quebec: Le Cercle Interdisciplinaire de Recherches Phénoménologiques (CIRP), l'Université du Québec.

——(2014). Qualitative inquiry in the history of psychology. *Qualitative Psychology 1*(1), 4–16.

Wertz, F. J., Charmaz, K., McMullen, L. M., Josselson, R., Anderson, R., & McSpadden, E. (2011). *Five ways of doing qualitative analysis: Phenomenological psychology, grounded theory, discourse analysis, narrative research and intuitive inquire*. New York: Guilford Press.

Westphal, M. (1998). *History and truth in Hegel's phenomenology*. Indianapolis: Indiana University Press.

Winnicott, D. W. (1965). *The maturational process and the facilitating environment*. New York: IUP.

Woolf, V. (1957). *A Room of One's Own*. New York: Harcourt Brace & World, Inc.

Wronka, J. (2008). *Human rights and social justice: Social action and service for the helping and health professions*. Thousand Oaks, CA: Sage Publications.

Zahavi, D. (2001). Beyond empathy: Phenomenological approaches to intersubjectivity. *Journal of Consciousness Studies*, 8, No, 5–7, 151–167.

Zaner, R. (2002). Making music together while growing older: Further reflections on intersubjectivity. *Human Studies 25*: 1–18, 2002. © 2002 Kluwer Academic Publishers. Printed in the Netherlands.

Zoloth-Dorfman, L. (1993). First, make meaning: An ethics of encounter for health care reform. *Tikkun*, *8*(4), 23–26.

Index

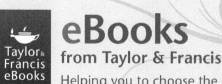
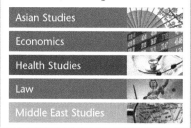